GOING THE EXTRA

Smile

GOING THE EXTRA

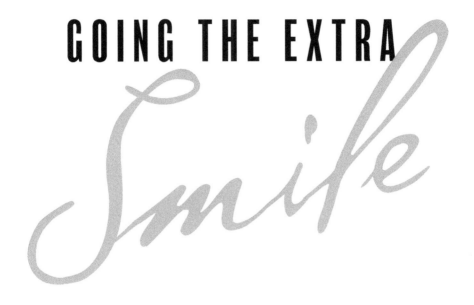

Smile

MERGING TECHNOLOGY AND EXPERTISE
FOR A LIFETIME OF SMILES

STEVEN J. MORAVEC
DDS, MS, MA

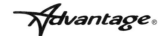

Published by Advantage, Charleston, South Carolina.
Member of Advantage Media Group.

ADVANTAGE is a registered trademark, and the Advantage colophon is a trademark of Advantage Media Group, Inc.

Printed in the United States of America.

10 9 8 7 6 5 4 3 2 1

ISBN: 978-1-64225-0039
LCCN: 2018955818

Book design by Carly Blake.

This publication is designed to provide accurate and authoritative information in regard to the subject matter covered. It is sold with the understanding that the publisher is not engaged in rendering legal, accounting, or other professional services. If legal advice or other expert assistance is required, the services of a competent professional person should be sought.

Advantage Media Group is proud to be a part of the Tree Neutral® program. Tree Neutral offsets the number of trees consumed in the production and printing of this book by taking proactive steps such as planting trees in direct proportion to the number of trees used to print books. To learn more about Tree Neutral, please visit **www.treeneutral.com**.

Advantage Media Group is a publisher of business, self-improvement, and professional development books and online learning. We help entrepreneurs, business leaders, and professionals share their Stories, Passion, and Knowledge to help others Learn & Grow. Do you have a manuscript or book idea that you would like us to consider for publishing? Please visit **advantagefamily.com** or call **1.866.775.1696**.

To my sister Patti, who taught me patience
and understanding at a young age.

TABLE OF CONTENTS

INTRODUCTION. 1

Changing Lives One Smile at a Time

CHAPTER 1. 7

Not Just Straight Teeth

CHAPTER 2. 15

Why Do I Need an Orthodontist?

CHAPTER 3. 27

The Earlier, the Better

CHAPTER 4 41

It's Never Too Late

CHAPTER 5. 49

New Options and Treatments

CHAPTER 6. 67

Getting from Here to There

CHAPTER 7 77
Life with Braces

CHAPTER 8 87
Clearing Up the Myths

CONCLUSION 99
A Great Smile to Last Forever

EPILOGUE 101
FAQ About Orthodontics

Changing Lives One Smile at a Time

Smile in the mirror. Do that every morning and you'll start to see a big difference in your life.

YOKO ONO

O rthodontics is my passion.

I know, most people think of passions as something they engage in outside of work—exercise, art, fishing, rescuing dogs. I'm not sure you'll hear investment bankers claiming that they can't get enough of interbank transfers, or plumbers waxing poetic about flush valves. But orthodontics is different. I can literally change someone's life for the better, while being able to engage in my lifelong love of technology and learning. How great is that?

Orthodontics, to me, is the most gratifying of any profession. Now, it may not be as exciting as acting or professional sports, or as dangerous as police work. It's not hard labor like coal mining, or as scientifically challenging as genetic research, but where else can I provide a great service to people—a lifelong smile—that enhances their lives and improves their overall station in life, while at the same time connecting with them on a personal level?

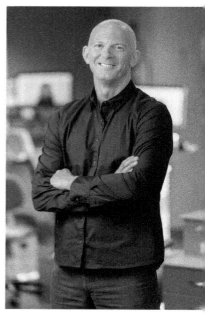

We often take our smile for granted. After all, we smile all the time; it's part of who we are. Smiling is so ingrained in human communication that new parents wait anxiously for that first smile. A parent smiles at their baby, and the baby smiles back. Suddenly, this needy baby connects and parent and newborn become one. Just look at how many countless smiles of toothless infants are posted on social media. That infant smile shows happiness, contentment and love. And you better believe on the other end of that smile are adoring parents smiling back. Now, once your teeth have come in, that smile really starts to shine, and it's that lifelong, beautiful bright smile that I, as an orthodontist, can help you get and keep.

Now, let's fast forward thirty to forty years and imagine you are in a business meeting. As a prospective client comes to you, what is the first thing you notice? Some might say, "hair" and, believe me, I understand that, but most will likely say it is the smile. We set people at ease with a smile and let them know we are happy to see them. When speaking on stage, we smile at the audience to try and connect. A smile is a universal language that says, "Don't be afraid. I'm friendly."

A smile is the gateway to your personality.

A smile is the gateway to your personality. When describing characters in books, authors invariably end up describing a smile. It could be a shy smile, a broad smile, a coy smile, a welcoming smile, a Miss America smile, or a tight-lipped smile. Less-savory characters might have sinister smiles or twisted smiles. It might be an insincere smile that doesn't reach the eyes. Describing the smile is describing the person and giving us clues to the person behind the smile.

Given all of this, who wouldn't want to be a professional that helps people get the smile they've always wanted? Orthodontics is the ultimate "helping" career.

I didn't grow up wanting to be an orthodontist. Like many fields, dentists and orthodontists tend to have a dentist or orthodontist in their family as a role model, just as actors' children often work in the entertainment industry, or engineers' children gravitate to STEM fields. However, there were no dentists in my family, so it wasn't on my radar as a child or teenager. In fact, and not surprisingly so, I wasn't a big fan of going to the dentist as a child.

But I did know I wanted to do something scientific or technical. I loved doing experiments, collecting bugs, building erector sets—all the things you associate with a curious kid. One of my middle school science teachers, Mrs. Atwood, encouraged my interest. I distinctly remember conducting an experiment in her class that involved a hamster in a maze. Looking back, I realize every kid in middle school must have done a similar experiment, where we recorded the times of mice and hamsters as they ran through mazes. I loved this experiment. I was fascinated by the whole process. I spent days tweaking variables—how many turns were in the maze, how many turns went right and how many left, where the hamster started, whether it had eaten or not—and testing to see how that changed the times. It was just the way my mind worked—and still works.

Another great influence on my young life and what probably pointed my future career into one helping people and improving lives was my sister Patty. Patty is five years younger than me. (I also have a brother, who is five years older than me, but no tears for the neglected middle kid, please.) Patty was born with Down Syndrome. Her generation of Down kids, born in the early 1960s, were the first to be raised at home instead of being institutionalized. As a child, I didn't realize how much patience and acceptance my parents had to have in raising Patty. For me, it was just natural to have a sister like Patty. But as I grew older, I came to see how my parents encouraged a culture of kindness and gentleness when it came to her. I believe this atmosphere of caring that I saw all around me as I was growing up helped develop my core values of understanding and empathy. I always want to do whatever I can to make life better for those around me.

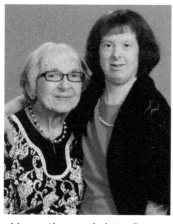

My mother and sister Patty.

Growing up with Patty helped make me who I am today. It not only made me come at the world from a place of kindness, but it encouraged me to find ways to enhance her life. With Down Syndrome, Patty developed not only mentally at a slower rate, but also physically, and she could not master the art of crawling on all fours. So I taught her how to scoot. She would sit cross-legged and then, with her arms fully extended against the floor, propel her butt and her body forward. As I recall, she became quite proficient.

So, when I began looking for a career that involved science and technology, but also involved helping people and enhancing their lives, I gravitated naturally to the medical field. As a kid, I wanted to be a veterinarian (so maybe not so much helping people as living things). It seemed to combine the technical and helping aspects I was looking for in a career. And how cool would it be to work with animals all the time?

That changed when I met my college girlfriend's father, who happened to be a dentist. I went to his office several times and saw him work. Not only was it in the medical field (check), it involved helping people (check) and was interesting enough to keep my attention long term (check). As a bonus, it also allowed him to set his own schedule, something I knew would work with my personality. I never saw myself as part of a large practice or tied to a hospital the way most medical doctors are. The medical field was also becoming very corporate and group practice oriented. Orthodontics was one of the last remaining areas in the medical field where you can have your own practice and make your own decisions. Being able to do my own thing appealed to my sense of independence—and to the fact that I really don't like being told what to do.

I also liked how personal orthodontics is. Instead of just seeing a patient once or twice a year, I see them frequently over one to two years and often see multiple family members for years on end. By running my own practice, I can make sure that each patient receives the totally individualized attention they deserve. Orthodontics is very one on one. I am the person providing my patients a great smile; I'm the person giving them healthy bites. When I see how happy they are with their smile, it is a very personal and direct reward.

Everyone deserves a great smile. Whether justified or not, in our society, study after study has shown that people with great smiles are judged to be more attractive and, hence, are thought of as being nicer, smarter, and better workers, among lots of other positive qualities. Having a good smile can make the difference between having the confidence at a job interview and not. It can make the difference between having someone accept a date and not—and thus maybe changing who you choose to share your life with. I'm proud to say that I've given thousands of people great smiles. When you multiply that by the thousands of personal interactions those patients have had over the years, I can see my work enhancing happiness and wellbeing in wider and wider expanding concentric circles. It makes me smile just to think of it.

By the time I finished college, I knew dentistry was the field for me. And it wasn't long before I knew I wanted to specialize in orthodontics. I'm precise and driven. Whether it is training for Ironman competitions, getting a master's degree in history, or tweaking treatment plans to give someone the perfect smile for their face, I don't stop until I've reached my goals. And if those goals involve tracking progress and challenging myself, so much the better.

Since becoming an orthodontist more than thirty years ago, I've treated thousands of patients. A lot of writers would end that line with "just like you." But no one is just like you. Orthodontics allows me to provide individualized care to each of my patients. Yes, there are some very common problems that result in very similar treatment plans. But I see the individual and love to make that little final tweak in each plan that makes the smile all your own. Orthodontics truly is gratifying—for me, but mostly for my patients. It really does change lives. Not many occupations give you that satisfaction day after day.

I decided to write this book to bring you into my world. I want everyone to know what orthodontics can do for you and/or your child, as well as how advances in technology are making obtaining that perfect smile easier than ever. Whether you need just a slight adjustment to your smile or a major realignment, there are processes now available that make the whole experience easier, less noticeable and less time intensive than ever.

Let me tell you about them.

CHAPTER 1

Not Just Straight Teeth

*Let us always meet each other with a
smile, for the smile is the beginning of love.*

MOTHER TERESA

I live quite a few miles from my office, so I'm on the expressway every work day. I'm a left-lane type of guy, and if the left lane is moving a bit faster than the speed limit, I'll also be going a bit faster than the speed limit. One day, I was driving to work and suddenly, I saw the flashing lights of an Illinois State Trooper behind me. "Not a great way to start the day" (that's the G-rated version), I grumbled as I pulled over. I rolled down my window and waited for him to approach, and I got my driver's license and registration ready. The trooper got to my car, leaned in the window, smiled, and said, "Do you recognize me?"

I quickly ran his face and the

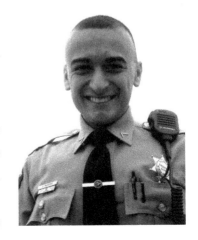

name on his badge through my memory bank and came up blank. I had to admit to him that I was sorry, but I just couldn't place him.

"I ran your plates when I was behind you and when I saw your name, I had to pull you over and thank you for my smile."

He had been one of my patients fifteen years before, and had stopped me just to thank me for his smile and tell me that he gets compliments on it all the time. What a great way to start my day! I snapped a quick cell phone photo of him standing next to the window, and I have kept it on my phone to this day.

We talk a lot about having a beautiful smile—and we should never discount how a great smile is good in and of itself—but having straight teeth is more than just personal vanity. Research has shown that having a pleasing smile can affect all areas of your life, from self-esteem to job prospects. One study has shown that those with straight teeth are viewed as happier, healthier, and smarter than those with misaligned teeth.[1]

One study has shown that those with straight teeth are viewed as happier, healthier, and smarter than those with misaligned teeth.

According to that same study, whether a person's smile and teeth are straight or crooked can have significant impact on his or her romantic success, because many Americans would not go on a second date with someone with crooked teeth. In fact, when it comes to attracting a possible mate on a dating site, those with straight teeth are much more likely than those with crooked teeth to get a date, based on their picture alone.

---

1   "First Impressions Are Everything: New Study Confirms People With Straight Teeth Are Perceived as More Successful, Smarter and Having More Dates," PR Newswire, April 19, 2012, https://www.prnewswire.com/news-releases/first-impressions-are-everything-new-study-confirms-people-with-straight-teeth-are-perceived-as-more-successful-smarter-and-having-more-dates-148073735.html.

And, of course, we all know the importance of first impressions. Another study even found that we make lasting judgments on a person's likeability just based on a quick glance of a photo.[2] The friendlier someone looked in a photo, the more the study participants thought they'd like them. Those test subjects who had been randomly assigned to look mean or unhappy in a photo were judged to have an unfriendly or less-likeable personality. Even after meeting the photo subjects in person one month later, this first impression held. No matter what a person's real personality was, if their photo was friendly, people thought they were nicer in person than were those who had had mean or unfriendly expressions in their photos.

A smile is one of the first things people notice and remember—for better or for worse—and nothing says "friendly" more than a great smile.

ECONOMIC BENEFITS

I recently had a father come in with his teenage son, who had gotten his braces off a few days before and was stopping by to pick up his retainers. I began my normal spiel. I asked him how he liked having his braces off and what his friends thought about his new smile. I then asked him if he knew the difference between buying something (like a car or shoes or a TV) and investing in something. I got the normal teenage answer—a shrug and a muttered response along the lines of, "Why are you asking me this?"

I explained that unlike something you buy that wears out, your smile is an investment that will increase in value through the years.

---

2   Gul Gunaydin, Emre Selcuk, and Vivian Zayas, "Impressions Based on a Portrait Predict, 1-Month Later, Impressions Following a Live Interaction," *Social Psychological and Personality Science* 8, no. 1 (2015), http://people.psych.cornell.edu/~pac_lab/pdf/Gunaydin,Selcuk,&Zayas,PortraitPrediction.pdf.

It is an investment in your future, and the first thing people notice about you after looking at your eyes. At this point, the dad jumped in and said, "Boy, you are so right."

The dad said he owns a software company, and he hires a lot of people. "A smile is the first thing I notice. When someone comes in for an interview, if you don't have a good smile or the type of smile that lets your personality shine through, that's one mark against you right there." It was nice to have him reinforce to his son—in very concrete terms—what I'd just told him.

This software company owner isn't alone in his assessment of the importance of a smile when applying for a job. More than 50 percent of people believe someone with crooked teeth would be less likely to land a job when competing with someone who has a similar skill set and experience and nice teeth. Americans also perceive those with straight teeth to be 58 percent more likely to be successful, as well as 58 percent more likely to be wealthy.[3]

SOCIAL BENEFITS

A while ago, I had a patient in her forties. She had immigrated to the United States from a rather undeveloped country, so she hadn't had the best dental care. She not only had to have her teeth and her bite aligned, but I also had to move her teeth into a better position, so her dentist could do some additional aesthetic treatment. She had a very plain look, and was quite reserved and a little timid when she came in. By the time I finished my treatment, and in combination with the work her dentist performed, she became a totally different woman. Hair done, makeup done, the beautiful smile, and, most

---

3   PR Newswire, "First Impressions Are Everything: New Study Confirms People With Straight Teeth Are Perceived as More Successful, Smarter and Having More Dates."

interestingly, a complete change in her personality, which was now outgoing and self-assured. All it took was a beautiful smile to give her the confidence to let her true self shine.

That happens a lot, particularly with my adult female patients. We always take photographs of our patients before we start treatment and, of course, we take photographs of them after they get their braces off or finish clear aligner treatment. Nine times out of ten, they have a new hair color and makeup, and a sparkle that was missing when they were embarrassed by their teeth.

Feeling a boost of confidence when you have a great smile is well warranted. A Harvard study found that people believe attractive people are more competent, warm, likeable, and trustworthy than those judged unattractive.[4] Although this study was focused on the use of cosmetics to enhance attractiveness, it isn't a huge stretch (or even a small stretch) to assume that an attractive smile will engender the same results in perception.

HEALTH BENEFITS

You probably intuitively know that a good smile makes people happier and more confident. All you have to do is think about how you feel when you know you look your best, and how you feel when you don't. But having straight teeth improves more than your social or economic health. It improves your physical health, as well. Once you begin thinking about it, I'm sure the reasons will be as obvious as those related to better social outcomes.

To begin with, straight teeth are easier to clean. This means you can keep tartar at bay and prevent cavities easier than if you are dealing

---

4   Nancy L. Etcoff et al., "Cosmetics as a Feature of the Extended Human Phenotype: Modulation of the Perception of Biologically Important Facial Signals," *PLoS ONE* 6, no. 10, (Oct. 3, 2011): https://doi.org/10.1371/journal.pone.0025656.

with overlapping teeth or wide gaps. Because you can control tartar better, you can prevent mankind's most common ailment—gum or periodontal disease. This is huge when it comes to overall health.

Gum disease has been linked with heart disease, strokes, and other chronic medical conditions.[5] The connection between gum disease and chronic health conditions seems to be inflammation—the body's natural response to an infection or injury. Gum disease develops when inflammation caused by tartar build-up and bacteria spreads to the tissues that support the teeth. It has been postulated that this inflammation is the beginning of the inflammation that spreads through the body, contributing to heart disease and other conditions. Eliminating or reducing gum disease, thus, could reduce heart-related problems.

While the effects of gum disease on your general health are still the subject of research studies, there is no doubt that properly-aligned teeth reduce the instances of cracked, broken, and worn teeth. Teeth were designed to mesh together with pressure spread relatively evenly across the top and bottom. Irregular teeth cause more pressure to be exerted on companion teeth than they were meant to withstand. Consequently, you may find yourself facing a broken tooth—and it always happens at the most inopportune time. Straightening and realigning those teeth will not only look better but will also save teeth that otherwise might be lost to disease, fracture, or wear.

Some patients with obstructive sleep apnea can also be helped by realigning teeth, correcting the bite, and correcting alignment of the jaw. We usually think of sleep apnea as being a condition associated with overweight adults. But we are finding that the condition is more

---

5   Julie Corliss, "Treating Gum Disease May Lessen the Burden of Heart Disease, Diabetes, and Other Conditions," *Harvard Health Publishing*, July 23, 2014, www.health.harvard.edu/blog/treating-gum-disease-may-lessen-burden-heart-disease-diabetes-conditions-201407237293.

common in children than we ever thought. Even in children younger than three years old. Lack of a good night's sleep can contribute to poor attention spans, poor school performance, poor growth, and poor social skills.[6] If the bite is corrected as a child, it can reduce mouth breathing, snoring, and in some cases, the sleep apnea itself. This can have a dramatic impact on these young children. Orthodontically repositioning the bite can also reduce the severity of sleep apnea as an adult. When dealing with either a child or an adult, repositioning the bite can provide an alternative to a CPAP machine, which is bulky and many find difficult to use. That being said, it is always necessary to contact and be assessed by a physician who specializes in sleeping disorder before undertaking orthodontic or dental procedures for sleep apnea.

Besides sleep apnea, straight teeth may reduce your risk of jaw and jaw joint disorders. Some studies have shown the jaw joint benefits from straight teeth, but just as many have shown that there is not a relationship. So the jury is still out on that.

BOTTOM LINE

A great smile with straight teeth improves health and happiness. There is no doubt about that. As an orthodontist, I love to hear the personal stories of how my work and my staff's work has paid off.

A great smile with straight teeth improves health and happiness.

Knowing that my patients will likely keep their teeth far longer than their grandparents did because their teeth will be easier to clean is gratifying, but hearing how their new smile has affected their day-to-day life is even better.

---

6   Brandon Peters, "Symptoms and Consequences of Sleep Apnea in Children," *Very Well Health*, Oct 5, 2017, www.verywell.com/what-are-the-consequences-of-sleep-apnea-in-children-3015069

One more example, if you will. One day, a woman in her mid-forties came in. Ten years earlier, I had treated her as an adult, and she was coming back in to have her retainer adjusted. I had also treated her two children a few years back. As she was getting ready to leave, she said, "Oh, I have to tell you. My son recently graduated from high school and in the senior yearbook he was voted 'Best Smile' in the class. Thank you for that." She then pulled out his senior picture to show me, and she was so proud of him having the best smile in the class.

I love my job!

CHAPTER 2

Why Do I Need an Orthodontist?

Everyone looks so much better
when they smile.

JIMMY FALLON

O ne of the first things I'm asked by parents, patients and even acquaintances is, "Why do I need to see an orthodontist?" This simple question really has two interpretations, and I often need to clarify before I can answer. They might be asking me if their teeth or bite need to be corrected. Or they might be asking if they really need an orthodontist, or if a general dentist could suffice. Or they might be asking both.

Let's start with the second interpretation of the question—can my general or family dentist take care of my orthodontic work?

ORTHODONTIST OR FAMILY DENTIST?

Your own family dentist is the expert in your overall dental and oral health. Their training and experience allows them to treat cavities, missing teeth, gum problems, and jaw problems, and most dentists today are the front line in the defense of oral cancers. Some general dentists might also be able to handle some minor orthodontic issues,

Orthodontics is much more than straightening teeth.

such as a slightly overlapped tooth or a small gap between the front teeth. But orthodontics is much more than straightening teeth. An orthodontist, as we discussed above, is an expert in the smile—and the smile is more than just straight teeth. A great smile is a balance between the teeth, the lips, and the gum line. With children and teens, facial growth and the changes that come with that must also be understood and added to the evaluation.

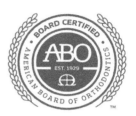

Look for this logo when choosing your orthodontist.

Becoming a specialist in orthodontics requires three years of specialized residency beyond the four years that all dentists spend in dental school. So, all orthodontists are dentists first, then go on for additional university training to become a specialist. It's a highly skilled specialty, the same way that oral surgery or endodontics (root canals) are specialties requiring years of additional training. During this training, orthodontists not only learn the mechanics of straightening teeth, but we spend numerous hours in class studying the interaction between the bones, teeth and facial muscles—how the jaw grows, how bone reacts to pressure, how to move teeth without damaging them, and other nuances unique to orthodontics. We also learn to take aesthetics into account. You don't want to just end up with straight teeth that look like a row of Chiclets. You want to end up with straight teeth that complement and conform with the shape of your lips and jaw.

Without this knowledge, mistakes can happen. It's not rare for me to reevaluate a patient who had first gone to their own dentist or another general dentist for orthodontic treatment. People who use their general dentist for orthodontics do so for a variety of reasons. Sometimes it's just because they are more familiar with their dentist and don't want to have to find a specialist. Sometimes, they think it will be cheaper (it rarely is). Sometimes, they think the issue is so minor that they don't need a specialist (it's hard for a non-orthodontist to really know if the issue is minor or not—what looks like a simple gap could actually be part of a bigger problem that will get worse as time goes on). Sometimes, it all works out fine. But sometimes, it doesn't.

My expertise as an orthodontist is especially important when evaluating and treating young children, preteens, and adolescents. Because their faces are growing and changing and baby teeth are falling out and adult teeth are coming in, it is a dynamic situation that requires a full and thoughtful assessment. There is usually a "best time" to begin orthodontic treatment in children, and we'll look at this in more detail later, but the "best time" is when we can be successful correcting the orthodontic problem in the least amount of time with the least amount of inconvenience to the patients and their parents.

Many dentists now offer Invisalign or other clear aligner systems and, in some cases, the standardized, templated process works fine. But even when the teeth look fine, an orthodontist might have been able to make them look better. Invisalign has given dentists the tools and an easily learned process to offer teeth-straightening services to patients with minor problems. But a dentist does not have the experience that an orthodontics specialist does to give you the *best* results. Dentists can become certified as an Invisalign practitioner after taking a two- or three-day course. They usually don't understand how the teeth move, or the particular sequence that should be employed when moving teeth. Most importantly, they often don't understand which types of cases work well with Invisalign and which don't. Most Invisalign cases treated by non-orthodontists are programmed by computerized software and aided by software technicians, with little input or critique by the practicing dentist. The average dentist who uses Invisalign treats fewer than ten cases per year, while most orthodontists, including myself, have treated hundreds of Invisalign and clear aligner patients in our careers, not to mention the thousands of patients treated with braces.

Not too long ago, I had a patient come in who had been working with her own dentist to realign crowded teeth. Unfortunately, in an effort to give the teeth more space, the dentist had pushed the teeth too close to the edge of the jaw bone, and a couple of teeth were becoming unstable. She was in danger of losing those teeth. Plus, the teeth just looked strange. Now this patient was in her early sixties and her chief complaint was that the women in her tennis group were starting to call her "Bucky Beaver" because of her teeth. As you can imagine, this comment was not exactly the type of "compliment" she was hoping for after spending thousands of dollars to get her teeth straightened. The teeth were straight for sure, but they were sitting on the outside of the jawline rather than in the middle, where teeth belong. I was able to realign the teeth and bring them back firmly into the jawline. But it took time, and while everything looks good at the moment, there is no guarantee that the most-affected teeth won't have issues in the future.

Being an orthodontist is similar to being an artist. Anyone can buy paints and apply them to a canvas. But the skill of a trained, experienced artist will make the difference between paint that just sits on a canvas and a piece of art that pulls you in and holds your attention. Think about paint-by-number kits. You will end up with an attractive painting when you are finished. You might even want to frame it and hang it on your wall. But it won't have that special aura or inner glow that artists bring to their work. Your smile is an investment in your future. You deserve to entrust it to a skilled specialist who can give you a smile that truly fits your face and speaks to who you are. You want someone who can give you that inner glow, not just color in the lines.

Orthodontists are focused on their niche in the oral health world. I spend hours reading journals to keep up on the newest innovations and spend many weekends at conferences and training sessions to make sure I'm offering my patients the best of what is available. I subscribe to an audio service that allows me to listen to taped summaries of journal articles while I'm driving to work or to one of my kid's athletic events. When I'm running or training for an Ironman triathlon, I let my mind wander and it often drifts to how I can incorporate these advances in my practice. I've had more than one eureka moment when I've just let my mind go where it wants to.

Keeping up with how the orthodontics is changing to make outcomes better for patients is almost a full-time job in itself and if I'm not putting in the time, I'm not really practicing modern orthodontics. I don't know how a general dentist could find the time to be on top of the advances in both the dental and orthodontic sectors, as well as be able to implement them into their everyday practice, while handling a caseload of patients. It is challenging enough for me—and orthodontics is my only job!

Besides best practices, I also make sure that I am using the most advanced

> **Besides best practices, I also make sure that I am using the most advanced technologies, so my patients benefit from the best and most-researched thinking.**

technologies, so my patients benefit from the best and most-researched thinking. Because orthodontics is all I do, I don't have to worry about anything except providing the best orthodontic care for my patients. My time isn't split between different specialties, so I can afford to dive deeply into the one I'm passionate about.

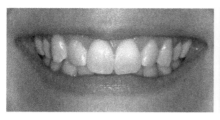

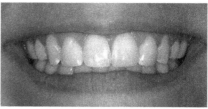

Treatment by a
non-orthodontist.

After I refined the treatment.
The smile line is better and the edge
of the teeth follow the lips.

For example, I make sure I have the technology skills to use the newest software to provide the best aesthetic outcome, as well as physical outcome. With a 3-D software program that we use in my office, I can superimpose the soft tissues (lips, nose and chin) over the hard tissues (jaw bones and the teeth). I then get a 3-D representation of how the patient will look and how moving the teeth will affect the appearance of the smile. This program also lets me factor in how the facial muscles are used to form the smile—everyone smiles differently, and I want to account for that. I can tweak the orthodontic plan until I get the optimal aesthetic look to go with the newly aligned teeth and bite. This all brings me back to my erector set and hamster maze days, when I could get lost in how small tweaks could change the entire integrity of a structure or the time it takes a rodent to transverse a maze. I'm a kid again, discovering how things work. And I love bringing that enthusiasm to my patients.

Being a specialist really makes a difference. I'm able to keep up on the cutting-edge advances occurring in the industry. I have the experience to look at a patient's mouth and quickly determine a treatment plan that will not only straighten their teeth, but also provide them with a smile that works with their face. Plus, I really like what I'm doing. The part of orthodontics I enjoy the most is meeting a new patient and their families and addressing their concerns and explaining treatment. A patient is an individual with an individual set of issues, and I enjoy using all the technology and information at my disposal to come up with the best treatment plan available for that particular patient.

Given how important your teeth are to your overall well-being, why would you take your teeth to a non-orthodontist to do orthodontic work?

The easiest way to find out if your orthodontic care provider is specialized is to ask this one question: "Are you a board-certified orthodontist who has two to three years of additional orthodontic training beyond dental school?"

DOES MY CHILD, OR DO I, NEED AN ORTHODONTIST?

Some people don't have to ask if their child needs an orthodontist. They can see the teeth are coming in crooked, or there is too much space, or even a tooth isn't coming in at all. You know if you or your child has crooked teeth; it's pretty obvious to everybody.

But there are many other teeth and bite issues that an orthodontist can pick up that aren't as obvious. We're picking up the subtler things, which can honestly be more important and sometimes more difficult to treat than are just crooked teeth.

One of the more important things we look at is your bite. Are the top and bottom teeth lining up the way they should? Is the lower jaw closing correctly—or is it jutting out or pulling in too much? Some over- and underbites are obvious, but many are subtler. The subtle ones are no less important than the obvious ones. A misaligned bite will be putting extra pressure on your teeth every time you chew, which over time can cause cracked teeth and can contribute to periodontal issues. We can avoid those complications by catching the misalignment early and correcting it while the jaw is still relatively malleable.

Parents often also miss the fact that adult teeth are going to be bigger than baby teeth, and your child's mouth needs room for those bigger teeth. I've heard many parents mention how happy they are that their four-year-old has a perfect smile with no spaces between their teeth. The problem with this is that when baby teeth line up perfectly against each other at four years old, as an eight-year-old, the larger adult teeth are going to overlap to all fit in the mouth. You actually want spaces between the baby teeth. If we see a child early enough, we can often use expanders and other appliances to open up those spaces, allowing permanent teeth to come into the mouth properly and possibly prevent the need for braces in the future. And if we can't prevent the need for braces, we can certainly make future issues less severe, and thus make the treatment plan shorter and simpler.

Your dentist is often the first person to mention the need for an orthodontic consultation. He or she sees thousands of mouths and usually knows when things don't look quite right. But even an experienced dentist can miss things, so you shouldn't assume that if nothing is said, everything is fine. To be safe, we suggest a screening exam at age seven. If there are obvious problems, earlier would, of course, be better, but at this age, adult teeth are beginning to emerge and how they will come in can be better assessed. I can see things that a dentist doesn't see when I look at a child, and we can begin drawing up a treatment plan if one is needed. Most children are not treated at these younger ages, but are placed in an observation program where growth and the eruption of teeth are monitored at regular six- to twelve-month intervals. That way, we don't miss the "best time" to start orthodontics, whenever that might be.

At these early ages, when adult teeth are just beginning to emerge, advanced technology helps us to intervene early, and mitigate future problems. We take high-tech, low-dose three-dimensional images, which can be manipulated in a variety of ways to give me an idea of how the teeth will look when they emerge. I have often seen problems that where missed with conventional 2-D x-rays. Corrective measures early on can save more extensive work down the line, so it's worth an assessment visit at age seven just to make sure everything is developing properly.

These early images also let us make sure all the adult teeth are growing correctly. It's not uncommon to see patients who are born without adult teeth. About 3 percent of the population are born with at least one missing tooth. Early screening lets us get a handle on this situation and make a plan to rectify it.

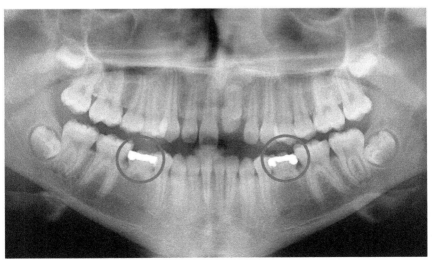

X-ray of a patient missing two adult teeth.

Conversely, 1 percent to 2 percent of the population is born with at least one extra tooth. We can usually pick those up on the 3-D image and have them removed before they impact the eruption and crowding of the other teeth. These are things that can often go undetected in a standard 2-D x-ray.

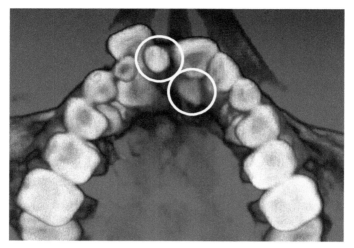

3-D image of a young patient with two extra teeth.

Another problem that needs to be treated early is an underbite, where the lower teeth are in front of the top teeth. Beginning treatment when the jaw is still forming makes it much easier to bring the jaw into alignment and correct the bite. Treatment of an underbite at six or seven years of age is optimal, as the jaw is still very malleable and can be repositioned with special orthodontic appliances. Once a child reaches the preteens years, correction of an underbite becomes much more difficult.

Adults usually know when they need an orthodontist. They often haven't liked their smile for years and now want to do something about it. Or they might have had braces as a child and their teeth have begun to shift. Another common reason for adults to visit the orthodontist is to prepare their teeth for dental cosmetic dental work, including crowns, bridges, and implants. We are often asked by a patient's family or restorative dentist to move teeth to allow more room for the proper placement of bridges and implants. Straighter, better-spaced teeth also provide a better foundation for veneers. For an adult, cosmetic concerns are often the main reason they seek orthodontic services. But just like for children and teens, straight teeth, a great smile, and an optimal bite go hand in hand with overall dental, oral, and general health.

EXPERIENCE MATTERS

Orthodontics is a skill that improves with practice. Whether you are looking for an orthodontist for yourself or your child, you will want to look for an experienced orthodontist for the best results.

> **Orthodontics is a skill that improves with practice.**

At this point, I've been in practice for more than thirty years and treated close to twenty thousand patients ranging in age from three to eighty-three. There isn't much I haven't seen. It's pretty rare nowadays for someone to come in and I think, "Wow, I haven't seen that in the last thirty years."

It's this experience that allows me to provide treatment plans with great outcomes, as well as know when they need to be adjusted because a tooth isn't moving as expected, or something else pops up that requires a detour in the plan. I've had enough experience to know that everyone is unique, and while there are general treatment plans that are used for specific issues, they need to be adjusted for each patient. I love doing that.

I've also have enough experience to be able to honestly tell you if you or your child really needs orthodontic treatment. Yes, this does happen quite often. One of the great sins of any medical field, including orthodontics, is treating a patient that doesn't need treatment or over-treating a patient that does. I know how a child's teeth will emerge. I've seen just about every permutation of that process. I can tell early on if the teeth that look a little misaligned today are going to straighten as others come in or are going to need help.

Relying on my experience will save you time and money in the long run, and secure better results.

And speaking of treatment, it's that part of the book where we move into more of the specifics involved in treating children and teenagers. Things have changed a lot since you were a child. Let me walk you through those advances.

CHAPTER 3

The Earlier, the Better

Wear a smile and have friends.

GEORGE ELLIOT

Most of you are undoubtedly familiar with braces. You may have even had them yourself or certainly had friends that had them. But I bet you were a teenager, or close to it, when you first started your treatment. Even if you never had braces yourself, I bet many of you think of braces as a teenage experience. You certainly don't think about them for kids who can't even read yet.

But things have changed since you were a teenager. Today, we know that some orthodontic concerns are better addressed at a much younger age when the teeth are still coming into the mouth and the jaw bones themselves are more pliable.

By "much younger age," I mean I like to see children for a screening consultation around the age of seven, or when their top two permanent teeth and the back six-year-old molars emerge. If baby teeth are obviously overcrowded, or if there is an obvious misaligned bite, it makes sense to see an orthodontist even earlier. I've worked with patients as young as three years old. One three-year-old came to me (well, his parent brought him) because his teeth and bite were so out of line that he was having trouble eating. My own daughter, Eva, was one of those patients. At age two-and-a-half, an upper baby front tooth was hitting behind the lower front baby teeth, causing the teeth to chip and become sore. She had some partial braces for about two weeks and the problem was corrected. She wasn't the best patient I ever had, but our father/daughter relationship survived the experience and she got to keep her blankie.

According to the American Association of Orthodontists, these are some red flags that a child may be a candidate for orthodontic care:

- Teeth coming in later or earlier than normal
- Crowded or misplaced teeth
- Protruding teeth
- Upper and lower teeth that don't meet, or meet in an abnormal way
- An unbalanced facial appearance, where the jaw or teeth are out of proposition to the rest of the face
- Difficulty chewing or biting
- Jaws that are too far forward or back
- Mouth breathing
- Thumb or finger sucking
- Biting the cheek or the roof of the mouth
- Sleep issues, including childhood sleep apnea and snoring
- Grinding or clenching of the teeth
- Difficulty speaking

Parents can often tell when a child's teeth are crowded, but sometimes it's hard for a parent to tell if the bite is off. A very common symptom of the back bite being off is a child's tendency to bite the inside of their cheek. This is usually caused by a "crossbite" of the back teeth, where top back teeth are inside the lower back teeth (the opposite of how the bite should be). When teeth and jaws are aligned correctly, you will rarely end up biting your cheek.

Now, I know most parents don't think about making an orthodontist appointment when their children reach first grade. It probably wouldn't cross their mind unless their pediatric dentist or family dentist says they should see an orthodontic specialist. But, actually, first or second grade is the perfect time to screen for minor and/or potentially major orthodontic issues.

Once those first adult teeth are in, I can pretty much map how much crowding the child is going to have and how the bite is going to develop. This is also an age to get a 3-D cone beam image, which we obtain on most of our initial consultation patients. The 3-D image is a remarkable tool, and I often diagnose problems that are frequently overlooked on individual, or even panoramic x-rays. The most common surprise is finding missing or extra permanent teeth. As mentioned in an earlier chapter, about 3 percent of people are born missing one or more adult teeth, and between 1 and 2 percent have extra teeth, not to mention the much more common finding of crowding and overlapped teeth that are developing hidden in the jaw bones.

For example, just a few days ago, as I was writing this book, a nine-year-old boy, Christian, came in for an initial consultation. I had treated his mother many years ago and an older brother a few years ago. His dentist, basing his opinion from an individual x-ray and what one could see clinically, told his parents that he thought he had an extra tooth and a missing tooth. Now this would be quite rare, as missing and extra teeth are genetic issues, and it would be unusual to have both genes in your family background. Nonetheless, that is what the family was told.

What did the 3-D image reveal? Well it showed not only one extra tooth, but a second one hidden behind his upper-right front tooth in the palate and no missing tooth. The tooth thought to be missing was actually so crowded it overlapped an adjacent tooth under the gums and wasn't clearly seen on the dentist's x-rays. Ideally, I would have liked to have seen Christian at age seven, and we could have started some preventative treatment earlier.

Now, why don't we see most of our patients at this young age? After all, in my office we don't charge for this initial exam. Well, old habits die hard, especially sometimes in dentistry. Yes, many years ago, orthodontists and dentists used to wait until all the adult teeth came in before we began thinking about orthodontic treatment. This was also the time when orthodontists requested the extraction of adult teeth on about 75 percent of the patients. Today, with early evaluations, that percentage of patients that require the removal of healthy adult tooth is less than 20 percent. Unfortunately, a lot parents and, remarkably, even some dentists still adhere to this 1970s mentality and still don't think about mentioning orthodontic consultations until all adult teeth are in. But we now know that if you wait that long, you might miss an opportunity to make the treatment easier and less time-consuming.

I recently saw fifteen-year-old identical twin sisters, Alyssa and Amanda. They were already sophomores in high school when they came to my office, and both still had a couple of baby teeth in their mouth, which is quite unusual at that age. Of course, their parents were told by someone or had it in their minds not to see an orthodontist until all the baby teeth were out and the adult were in. Well, they still had baby teeth because the adult eye-teeth (cuspids) were not coming in at the right angle to eat away the root of the baby eye-teeth, allowing them to fall out. If Alyssa and Amanda had been evaluated at a much younger age, corrective measures could have been taken. Now, because they have impacted cuspids, their treatment will be much more complicated and time consuming than it would have been with an earlier assessment.

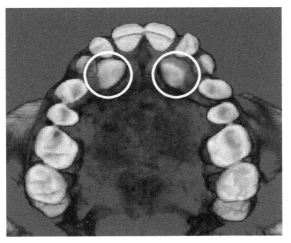

3-D image of a upper impacted canine (eye-teeth) coming in at very unfavorable angles.

They are going to need a minimum of two-years of orthodontic treatment and I'll need the help of an oral surgeon to "expose" the impacted cuspids to help me bring them into proper alignment and give Alyssa and Amanda the great smiles they want. Remember, Alyssa and Amanda are in the middle of their sophomore year in high school. Now, I'm not an expert on the teenage psyche, but I can be pretty sure that most teenage girls (and boys, for that matter) would rather not have braces for their homecoming dances, junior and senior proms, and—most of all—graduation. Their senior yearbook pictures might even memorialize the fact that they had braces from the middle of their sophomore year through senior year. If we'd seen these kids for an early assessment with a 3-D image, we would have been able to prevent a lot of that work, and certainly would have had them in and out of braces much earlier than their senior year in high school.

At a first- or second-grade age, there are often issues obvious to the trained eye of an orthodontist that a parent, or even some dentists, wouldn't notice. Parents are often thrilled to have a child with baby teeth that butt up against each other in a perfectly straight line. While this smile looks great in preschool pictures, it doesn't bode well for the future. We often hear parents say, "My kid's baby teeth were so straight and perfect. What happened? Now they look terrible."

Well, what usually happens is that much larger adult teeth are replacing the smaller baby teeth and, unless there were spaces between the baby teeth, there is often a crowding problem. Believe me, parents, you don't want perfect baby teeth—you want nice spaces between them. However, if we see these kids early enough, we can often prevent the overcrowding of adult teeth, so the permanent teeth look just as great as the baby teeth did.

Other problems an orthodontist might pick up in an early-age consultation besides missing teeth, impacted teeth, and crowded teeth include unusual growth patterns in the jaw—which will eventually become obvious in overbites or underbites, i.e., upper and lower jaws that don't meet correctly—or problems due to thumb, finger, or lip sucking. One of the things that separates orthodontists from your dentist is our training in how the bones in the face, including the jaw, develop and interact with each other. By the age of seven, I can usually spot issues in the growth patterns or bone formation and start correcting or observing the issues I see to avoid potential future problems.

Now, that all being said about wanting to see children for their first orthodontic visit at about age seven, it is important to realize that most children this age *do not* need actual orthodontic treatment. This first meeting is usually more of a preventative consultation, as well as a chance for the orthodontist and child to get comfortable with each other.

When you come in with your younger child for this first meeting and after I assess their photographs and 3-D images along with a clinical examination, it is most likely that we'll place your son or daughter on a six- to twelve-month recall program to observe the eruption of adult teeth and the growth of the jaws. I can also give you a fairly accurate estimate of when your son or daughter would be best treated based on the timing of the eruption of their adult teeth and their jaw development. This can be a valuable aid in planning future insurance and budgeting needs.

I actually recommend an early interceptive or "first-phase" of orthodontic treatment in only about 25 percent of the younger patient I see. The first phase plan might include braces on just a few teeth, such as protruding front teeth; an expander to widen the jaw; a simple holding arch or space maintainer to allow open paths for emerging adult teeth; or devices to help patients with thumb- and finger-sucking habits, or with sleep apnea; or a combination of all the above. This early treatment typically lasts less than a year, after which we would have periodic appointments to track how the adult teeth are coming in and evaluate the need for braces or clear aligners later in the preteen or teen years.

A second phase, which normally includes full braces or a clear aligner system like Invisalign or SureSmile aligners, would begin, on average, in middle school. Parents sometimes wonder if the child will simply outgrow the issues, but jaw, bite, and overcrowding problems usually do not take care of themselves. It's best to have them assessed as early as possible. This is one of the most pervasive myths we deal with, and I talk more about it in Chapter 9, where I examine popular orthodontic myths.

GETTING DOWN TO THE NITTY GRITTY

You are probably wondering exactly what issues I've been alluding to when I talk about things we can—and should—treat at a young age. After more than thirty years working with children, I know there are several issues that can be helped tremendously with early intervention.

Jaw development is a primary concern at this age. Because young children are growing so fast and their bones are still relatively malleable, we can often help guide a wayward jaw into its proper alignment before it affects a child's teeth or facial structure. Doing so early will prevent more severe problems later on.

Another issue we often see at an early age is overcrowded or overlapping baby teeth. If they are overcrowded at this age, there is no doubt they will be doubly overcrowded when the adult teeth all come in. We can use an expander to widen the palate and jaw line to give the teeth more room, and hopefully lessen the overcrowding as larger teeth emerge. We can also use spacers or partial braces to help keep the gaps created by lost baby teeth wide enough to accommodate the new teeth coming in. It's a passive treatment that lets us hold space open so teeth can come in straighter than they would without assistance. Additional treatment will still probably be needed later, but it is likely the issues will be less severe and treatment time shorter if we can attack the overcrowding early.

Expanders, which we use to widen the palate, are part of a more active treatment plan. Widening the palate in younger kids is not only necessary to make room for adult teeth to come in straight and provide a more aesthetic appearance, but it can also help kids who have breathing problems. A lot of kids with very narrow pallets have restrictive nasal breathing, so they tend to snore. Sometimes, they even have sleep apnea. Poor sleep habits can result in poor school performance and slower physical development. I often have parents tell me that they are not only happy with how much better their child's teeth look after early orthodontic treatment, but now they're sleeping better, as well. They're not breathing through their mouth, they're breathing through their nose. That's always a nice message to get. Orthodontic treatment of pediatric sleep apnea patients is new and rewarding part of modern day orthodontics.

Parents often ask if the jaw will simply grow larger on its own to accommodate the larger teeth. Of course, the jaw continues to grow past age seven or eight, but it grows in a specific way. It doesn't get wider; it grows in length. So, if you have an eight-year-old or a nine-year-old with crowded front teeth, the jaw isn't going to widen in that area. It grows in the back, where the molars and, eventually, the wisdom teeth come in. Without the use of expanders and other devices, the jaw will not widen on its own to provide room for crowded teeth.

Another major issue is impacted teeth. The most common teeth to be impacted are the top eye teeth, or the canine teeth (remember our identical twin sisters, Alyssa and Amanda, from a few pages ago), but I've seen, at one point or another, that any of the adult teeth can be impacted. No matter which teeth are involved, it is very important to catch them early.

These impacted teeth are easily diagnosed with a 3-D cone beam image, and I can recommend proactive treatment to help these impacted teeth come down on their own. This usually involves the early removal of some baby teeth and the placement of a passive holding arch. It becomes a much more difficult problem to correct when we see a teenager with impacted teeth, so we want to avoid that if possible.

One question we often get from parents is, "Will my child need to have teeth pulled?" As we stated earlier, most of these parents remember tooth extraction as being a normal part of orthodontics. Of course, it depends on the child, but it's not nearly as common as it was thirty or forty—or even twenty—years ago. Back then, probably 75 percent of orthodontic patients had teeth pulled. Now, because we can move teeth earlier to make room for emerging adult teeth, we probably see extractions in less than 20 percent of our patients. That being said, it's definitely necessary in certain situations, and that's where the expertise of an experienced orthodontist is important. If the teeth are very crowded and you attempt to straighten the teeth simply by pushing them to the side and forward, you can actually push them too far. They have to go somewhere. You can only push teeth out to the side so much before you run out of the bone and the gums. After all, the teeth need to be positioned in the bone and gums properly to insure their life-long health. As an orthodontist, I know if there is enough bone to move the teeth out, or if extracting teeth to make room is the better option. Most often, early intervention provides a better outcome than waiting until all the teeth have come in. Sometimes, if we pull the baby teeth early, before adult teeth emerge, we give those permanent teeth a place to come, rather than having them come in crooked and crowded. This means that less involved treatment will be needed down the road.

It also makes sense to fix problems early that might cause teasing at school or embarrass the child, such as protruding front teeth or front teeth that are in substantially out of line. A short-term treatment plan, often with just some partial braces for a less than a year, can straighten teeth for a better aesthetic appearance. I don't think we should ever discount how important it is that young children feel good about their appearance. This is the time when self-confidence and how they interact with the world is cemented. We want them to feel confident when they smile, and not hide their teeth out of embarrassment.

Parents sometimes don't realize how crooked teeth are affecting their child. Or they might know they need to get to an orthodontist, but they get busy and think they will do it next month, or the next month, or the next year. Before you know it, the child has all of their adult teeth, and we have a much more severe problem.

I just had a patient recently, who is a freshman in high school. His mom was kind of embarrassed because I had treated her daughter at a much younger age a few years ago, but in her own mind, braces were a high school thing. Her daughter was telling her she should take her son in for a consultation, but she procrastinated and procrastinated. Now, he has to go through two years of high school with braces on when, if we had seen him earlier, we could have lessened the time in braces, plus we could have given him that smile of confidence that is important during the challenging years of adolescence.

I think if parents remember that baby teeth are the foundation for the adult teeth waiting to emerge, they will understand better why early treatment—or at least an early consultation—is so important. The more we can do to shore up that foundation, the better the outcomes for the adult teeth.

PRETEENS AND TEENS

Although I strongly believe the best time to start seeing an orthodontist is when the child is in first or second grade, as stated earlier, most children don't need

> I strongly believe the best time to start seeing an orthodontist is when the child is in first or second grade.

early treatment and are best treated when most, if not all, adult teeth are in, which is typically in the middle school years, realistically, between the ages of eleven and fourteen. Now, what do I mean by "best treated?" Well, for me, "best treated" means correcting any smile, alignment, and bite issues, but also correcting the problem in the *least amount of time* with the fewest number of visits to my office. That's why we have adopted cutting-edge technologies like the previously mentioned 3-D images and, as we will discuss later, the SureSmile digital system and clear aligners such as Invisalign.

Braces used to be most common in the later teen years but moving the treatment timeframe up a few years makes a lot of sense. A middle-schooler is old enough to have most, if not all, of his or her adult teeth, but still young enough where I can modify the natural growth of the jaws to correct bite problems.

In general, patients at this age are also old enough to be compliant with the plan, to wear appliances if needed, and provide a high level of hygiene, so the teeth and gums are protected. It is important that these young teens and preteens be active participants in their treatment. Some parents express concern whether their son or daughter will be responsible and do the things needed to take care of their braces or wear their aligners. For the vast majority of patients, the answer is a resounding "yes." I also like to remind these concerned parents that, hey, in few years, you are going to be handing over the keys to the family car to these kids, so best they learn to take on some responsibility sooner rather than later.

There was a time, in the now distant past, when kids with braces were teased because they were different. Today, it seems every eighth grader has braces, so having brackets and or aligners is really no big deal. I don't think kids are teased by being called "metal mouth" any more. Heck, there would be more kids to tease than there would be kids to tease them. This certainly illustrates just how commonplace braces are in the eleven-to-fourteen-year-old age bracket. Some might even argue that it is the kids without braces who are the outliers.

Although braces for older teens have become much less common than they were before, there are still some times when we need to wait. We don't need to wait for all of the adult teeth to come in, but we *do* need a good foundation. Kids with very late-forming teeth might be closer to fifteen than thirteen when they start treatment. And, as mentioned before, sometimes parents just procrastinate. We can still correct problems in high school age kids, but let's not wait that long if we don't need to. But, if you do wait, even if you wait until you are well into adulthood it's never too late to begin orthodontic treatment.

THE BOTTOM LINE

It's always best to have an earlier orthodontic assessment. If treatment is needed, then sooner is often better than later. Optimal timing is going to be based on when the teeth are ready, not the patient's age. So, get your first-grader in to see an orthodontist and let an expert decide if the time is right. You'll never regret it.

CHAPTER 4

It's Never Too Late

Nothing you wear is more
important than your smile.
CONNIE STEVENS

A t the end of the previous chapter, I said it's never too late to begin orthodontic treatment, and I meant it. We usually think about orthodontics as a rite of passage for a preteen or teen, but I've treated patients in their sixties, seventies, and even a few into their eighties. In fact, more and more adults seek and commit to orthodontic treatment than ever before. Adults now make up about 30 percent of all orthodontic patients.[7] That means you won't have to feel like Gulliver among the Lilliputians when you are sitting in my waiting room. There are sure to be other adults sitting there as well, and they won't be parents (though I have treated many parents and their children at the same time).

One of the reasons that more adults are getting braces or clear aligners well into their retirement years is simply that more adults

---

7   "Adults are seeking orthodontic treatment in record numbers," Dental Tribune, April 29, 2016, https://us.dental-tribune.com/news/adults-a.

are getting orthodontic treatment. The more adults that seek orthodontic treatment, the more acceptable it becomes. It's a wave that has reached a tipping point, where it is no longer strange to see a work colleague or your aunt in braces. Twenty or thirty years ago, it would have been quite rare to see to celebrities and sports stars such as Tom Cruise, Faith Hill, Justin Bieber, Danny Grover, Faye Dunaway, Draymond Green, and Dwight Howard sporting braces and wrinkles, as they have recently. In this age of adult self-improvement and life-long health, orthodontic treatment is just one more tool in the toolbox to help you reach your goals.

Most common reasons for adults to have orthodontic treatment:

- They simply want to look better
- People are living and working longer and see orthodontics as an investment in their future
- Clear aligners such as Invisalign and SureSmile aligners don't require braces at all
- Innovations have made metal braces cheaper, less noticeable and more efficient than ever before
- Lingual (behind the teeth) braces that can't be seen
- Had orthodontics as children or teens and they need a tune-up
- Could not afford them before and now they can
- Want to improve dental health
- Need to move teeth to prepare for dental restorative work

There are as many reasons to get braces as an adult, as there are to get them as a child. One difference, however, is that as an adult, you get to control how much work you want done and when you want to start. As a child, you have to rely on your parents to make those decisions.

Many adults have lived with crooked teeth or an uneven bite their entire life. They've never been happy with their smile, but they never thought they could do anything about it and for whatever reason, orthodontics wasn't available to them as children. Maybe it was an economic issue or, perhaps, they lived in an area or country not serviced by orthodontics or quality dental care. Or maybe they had braces as a child, but their teeth shifted in their adult years. This is not at all unusual. For some, crooked teeth are just part of who they are, and they don't think about it that much. For others, they are a major embarrassment that negatively affect their self-confidence, and their ability to be as social and successful as they could be. Straight teeth are also easier to clean, as already mentioned, and thus more likely to resist periodontal problems (loss of bone and gums that support the teeth).

At this point, I'd like to discuss Su Lin. Su Lin came in to my office for her first orthodontic visit at age forty-six. She had immigrated to the United States in her early twenties and worked as a paralegal for a local attorney. I had treated this attorney's children, and she had encouraged Su Lin to see me. Su Lin was shy, reserved, and, above all, did not like to smile. The dental care in her country of birth was not the best, and she had mismatching crowns on a few upper front teeth and pretty severe crowding of her lower teeth. She agreed to be treated, but because she was so soft spoken I didn't know if she was excited about our adventure together or not. Slowly over time, as she came in for her six-week visits and her teeth started to align, her personality came out. After never saying more than a few words to anyone during her first visits, I noticed her having long conversations with her patient manager and even with me! By the time I had finished her SureSmile braces treatment sixteen months later and, in conjunction with her family dentist who did a great job on her mismatched crowns, she was a totally different person and definitely not afraid to smile. Of course, like many of my adult female patients, the day she got her braces off saw her come in with a new hair style and makeup. A few others have even come in with a new boyfriend.

People don't die at sixty with rotten teeth any more. Dentistry and access to modern dentistry, along with fluoridated water and an emphasis on healthy gums, means that most people can maintain their one set of adult teeth for a lifetime. I know my own grandmother, who was born in 1900, lost all her teeth and wore dentures well before the end of her life. My own mother, now in her nineties, has lost only two teeth. We are living much longer and want to preserve our natural teeth. It used to be rare to meet people in their nineties. Now, I bet you know at least one person, if not several, well into their nineties and maybe even over age one hundred. Because we expect to live healthy productive lives for several more decades, patients in their forties, fifties and sixties see braces as an investment in their future. My oldest two patients were in their early eighties. One was a retired professor and the other a many-times-over grandmother. They were both thrilled with the results and couldn't stop smiling. I expect someday to have a patient even older. Adult patients are prioritizing their smiles. Being able to greet the world with a smile they are proud of is what they want and deserve.

While simple aesthetics is often reason enough to invest in orthodontics as an adult, there are also valid oral and overall health reasons to do so. When your teeth overlap or have come in at odd angles, food is hard to remove, and plaque and tartar can build up. This build-up of plaque and tartar is the main cause of periodontal and gum disease, which is the leading cause of tooth loss in adults. Teeth that don't meet properly will also wear down unevenly, causing irregularities and damaging wear of tooth enamel. None of this is good, and all can be mitigated or even prevented with straight teeth and a well aligned bite.

Looking at one's overall or systemic health, several studies have shown that there could be a relationship between periodontal disease and heart disease and possibly other overall health issues, as mentioned in the second chapter. While this is still a subject of clinical research, the thinking is that anything that causes an inflammatory response in the body (and this is what periodontal disease is) can cause the body to react in unhealthy ways. This becomes more of a reality as we age, making the investment in straight teeth even more of a priority. When we are young, we might hear that gum disease can impact overall health. But at that age, it's just theoretical. When you reach your forties and fifties, it becomes more real, and you begin to take notice of lifestyle changes that can improve health. Straightening your teeth is one thing you can do that doesn't involve changing eating or exercise habits. It's a passive intervention that can pay off in big ways.

So that's enough about systemic health and periodontal disease. Let's look at why most adults seek orthodontic care—they want a great smile to look better. In some ways, orthodontics is no different than a myriad of things we do to look and feel younger. No different than wrinkle cream, Botox, hair implants, tummy tucks, makeup, six-minute abs, hair dying, and large font print so you don't have to wear your reading glasses. The difference is, however, is that it will last a lot longer and, as we stated early in the book, the smile is one of the first things a new person first notices about you.

Now let's pretend, or maybe you don't have to pretend, that you're a divorced father or mother of three children and the last one is just about to the leave the house. Besides saying "yippee" to yourself, you have decided it's time to take care of yourself again. You've also been seeing all these ads online and on TV for mature (people over forty) dating sites. Now you have three choices for that profile photo. One, do what most people do and put up a photoshopped image. But you have too much integrity for that. Two, put one up where you're not smiling. But then you'll come across as smug and/or dull. Three, decide you want to have a great profile photo with a great smile and visit your local orthodontist and start Invisalign or SureSmile aligners treatment.

Advances in orthodontic technology like Invisalign and SureSmile (more on these later) have also been a factor in the increasing numbers of adults willing to undergo orthodontic therapy. We are able to accommodate just about any level of treatment with much more comfortable and less noticeable options than you remember as a child. All brackets now are incredibly small. If you opt for clear ceramic brackets, they are nearly invisible. We can put brackets behind the teeth (lingual braces) if you want a totally invisible look. No matter what type of brackets you decide on, we can use our SureSmile system to reduce the amount of time needed for treatment. (Again, I'll be explaining the SureSmile system in more detail in a later chapter.) We can often take a standard sixteen-month treatment plan and reduce it to eight or nine months using SureSmile. And, of course, for many types of orthodontic problems, we can use clear, removable aligners such as Invisalign or SureSmile aligners. The popularity of Invisalign and the mainstream marketing of that treatment technique has greatly increased public awareness of adult orthodontic treatment.

When treating adults, some factors come into play that are not generally seen in children and adolescents. First, your overall dental health and previous or anticipated dental treatment is important. Adults have crowns, bridges, implants, missing teeth, root canals, and some may have had gum or jaw issues that are rarely seen in children or teens. A very common reason adults seek orthodontic therapy is for me to prepare and position the teeth so their family or restorative dentist can complete their work in the best possible way. As an adult, you have more of a say in your treatment desires than a child. You may not want to devote the time and money for a complete, ideal correction. You may only want to have straight teeth and a better smile. That means you might opt for a shorter treatment plan and just straighten the front teeth or straighten the teeth but not try to achieve a perfect bite. As long as you are aware of the possible drawbacks to "partial treatment," this is a valid approach.

In general, just about anyone who wants orthodontic treatment as an adult can have it. Age in and of itself is no barrier. Remember, my oldest patients have been in their eighties. We can work with dental crowns, implants, veneers,

Just about anyone who wants orthodontic treatment as an adult can have it.

and missing and worn teeth. The most important thing for adult patients is to have healthy gums and bone supporting your teeth. If you've had periodontal (gum and bone) disease before and it has been successfully treated by your dentist or periodontist, you can also have a successful orthodontic experience. If you have active periodontal disease, that must be addressed first, prior to starting to move your teeth with orthodontics. The jawbone, teeth, and gums all need to be healthy to support braces. If someone with gum or bone disease wants to straighten their teeth, we have them work with a dentist or periodontist to clear up any problems. Then we can proceed with getting them the smile they want.

Deciding to get your teeth straight and obtaining a great smile is only the beginning of the process. In the past, all we could offer were ugly metal bands and wires. We now offer a wide variety of choices (and bands are no longer one of them), including mix-and-match options. I'll outline the pros and cons of each option in the next chapter.

Before we leave this chapter on adult orthodontic treatment, I'd like to relate one more story that is very common. Theresa had braces as a teen about twenty-five years ago. She wore her retainers faithfully for quite a while, even through college, but life took over, and she wore them less and less often. That, combined with a natural tendency for our teeth to crowd in our thirties and forties, caused a pretty significant shift in her bottom front teeth and some minor "relapse" in the upper front teeth. Her original orthodontist had done an outstanding job and her back bite was still nearly perfect. She came into the initial consultation visit fearing the worst and remembering only the trying aspects of her childhood orthodontic experience—braces for a couple years and a $5,000 to $6,000 payout. Theresa was pleasantly surprised when I told her she did not need a complete set of braces. Her back bite was great, and we only had to align the upper and lower front teeth. I prescribed a clear aligner treatment that took four months for the upper teeth and ten months for the lower teeth at a cost of several thousand dollars less than full treatment.

CHAPTER 5

New Options and Treatments

---

*Always wear a smile because
you never know who is watching.*
GRACIE GOLD

---

et's reminisce for a few minutes. A lot of you probably remember having braces as a kid, or certainly having friends who had braces. Nearly everyone remembers worrying before the braces were placed and being self-conscious that first day. Braces in those days were pretty hard to miss. Prior to the mid-1980s, a wide metal band was placed on each tooth. It was so big that it pretty much took up the whole tooth. Between the bands and the thick wire that ran through them, there was a lot of metal in the mouth, hence the terms "metal mouth" or "brace face," that we now only hear in period pieces set in the sixties or seventies, but never on the playground today. Everything—bands and wires—were always silver, so everyone's mouth looked the same.

Besides lacking an aesthetic appeal, braces during that time were uncomfortable to wear, and involved an uncomfortable (some would say painful) process to put on. Orthodontists would start by taking impressions with a tray of sticky goop that had to get firm in the patient's mouth for a couple minutes. Gagging was often a problem. Then we would set up several appointments to put on the bands. They were very uncomfortable to put on because we had to jam these little metal bands in between each tooth. If teeth were particularly tight, we might start by forcing spacers between the teeth and waiting a week or so to work the bands on. Each band took a long time to place, and it usually took several appointments to put all the bands on the teeth. Add onto this the fact that the patient had to come in every two to four weeks for about two years or more to have the wires replaced and tightened, and you have quite a commitment in time.

The world of orthodontics has changed dramatically since then and continues to evolve. Let's start with the preparation. Instead of bad-tasting impression goop, we can now usually get all the models of the teeth we need via 3-D scanning. The scanner basically produces thousands of little images that are combined to produce a 3-D computer model. These 3-D computer models can also be made into physical models with 3-D printing. These scanned images are not only easier on the patient, but they are much more precise than models made from impression trays, meaning we can develop better treatment plans.

Then we move to the braces themselves. Instead of wide bands, today's metal braces consist of small brackets that are glued onto the teeth with a resin. Most patients don't even feel them going on. We'll discuss other options beside regular metal braces shortly.

You might also remember the headgear or night brace that would go around the back of the neck or over the head. This was used to push teeth back and adjust the bite. Slumber parties in movies set in the sixties always have at least one character wearing this well-known piece of equipment. In the future, movies set in the 2000s will never include this device. It's not that it doesn't work. It's actually very effective—when worn as prescribed. But today's patients are so active that it's hard to get them to wear headgear enough to make a difference. Because we have other effective ways to get the same results, the famous headgear has fallen into the same oblivion as rotary phones, cassette tapes, and road maps.

The story of the headgear is really the story of orthodontics today—things that worked well in the past have been replaced by something better and more in tune with today's time-crunch society. In order for the headgear to work, the patient must wear it. This can create a voluntary compliance issue. Kid's might go to bed with it, but they could take it off in the middle of the night. Their parents didn't know and since it was only effective if it was being worn, treatment often failed. Because of these types of issues, not just with headgear but with orthodontics in general, there has been a move to what's called non-compliance therapy. In other words, things that are attached to the teeth or the wires that work on their own without patient input or patient cooperation. It makes it easier for everyone—patient, parents, and orthodontists—as well as resulting in better and faster outcomes.

And remember the once-a-month appointments for two years or more that we mentioned earlier, and that you might remember from having braces as a child? Those appointments are now more likely to be every six or eight weeks for sixteen months. That means instead of twenty-four appointments, we are looking at eleven or twelve appointments. That's quite a savings in time. I can't think of one patient or parent who would like to spend more time in my office (though it's very nice) rather than on the soccer field or at a friend's house.

A lot of these improvements in patient comfort and general outcomes is driven by the researchers at the orthodontic schools, as well as by manufacturers, who realize they can make small brackets that work just as well as broad bands, or digital scans that work better than impression trays. It's up to each orthodontist to keep abreast of the newest trends, which is where experience comes in. New orthodontic methods and materials come out frequently. Many are based on good research, but some are more designed to enhance the bottom line of businesses rather than promote patient health. I feel my thirty years of experience goes a long way in determining which innovations should be adopted to improve the patient experience and create better treatment outcomes.

> **It's up to each orthodontist to keep abreast of the newest trends, which is where experience comes in.**

There are certain principles of orthodontics—how the teeth move, how the bone forms, what forces we use, how orthodontic specialists understand the growth and development of the face—that are constant, and it doesn't really matter what you use or what you've been sold. You still have to adhere to those biological principles that allow us to move teeth. This knowledge really separates a trained board-certified orthodontic specialist from dental practitioners, who may just dabble in braces or Invisalign.

Every office has computers, at least we sure hope they do. (Note to patient: one clue that you are not in an office that is even close to updated technology is if they are still writing your treatment notes on a paper chart.) But today, modern orthodontics goes far beyond digital treatment notes and payment systems. I have always prided myself on adopting the best proven and most modern technology. For example, we started using low-dose digital x-rays when almost every other office I knew was still using a darkroom to develop old film x-rays. Remember the days when your dentist would hold the x-rays up to a light or window to read them? Now, we have 3-D imaging that gives much information than did old 2-D x-rays. I know when people come into my office for second opinions, and we show them the 3-D image, they still often say, "Oh, we've never seen anything like that before."

The other big thing that's changed is the wires. It's the wires that are moving the teeth. The braces are just little handles. We now have super-elastic wires, which can bend and come back to their shape easily and with less discomfort to the patient. Before the development of these wires, the patient had to go in every four weeks because the orthodontist had to bend the wire to move the teeth. Now, with these super-elastic alloy wires, the length of time can be extended a bit, sometimes every six weeks, sometimes every eight weeks, so the patients don't have to come into the office as often as they used to.

TODAY'S ORTHODONTIC TREATMENT CHOICES

Patients now have a lot more choices than they did even ten years ago. Depending on the severity of the issue and personal preference, patients can choose metal braces, ceramic braces, or lingual (behind the teeth) braces. Of course, for many patients, the treatment choice they prefer is clear aligners, Invisalign being the name that is most well-known. Or they can mix and match. I work with my patients to choose the best option, given their needs. No matter which type of braces the patient chooses, we usually add the SureSmile treatment process into the plan, which results in a much more precise outcome in 25 to 35 percent less time.

Although new hardware and innovative processes now give patients more choices than ever, metal braces are still the most commonly used method of straightening teeth, especially for children.

As mentioned earlier, metal brackets are glued to the teeth in a relatively short and painless process. First, we polish and dry your teeth. Then we use a really mild acid to microscopically roughen up the surface of the enamel. A composite, which is similar to the product your dentist would use for a white filling, attaches the braces to the teeth. All we have to do is press them on. It's so easy that patients don't even feel anything but the slightest pressure. Less than if you just pressed your finger against your tooth. Once all the brackets are attached, we harden the adhesive by shining an LED light on the brackets for a few minutes. We can usually put on a full set of braces, top and bottom, in about forty to fifty minutes, as opposed to before, when it would take three or four appointments to complete the job.

One of the fun innovations that has occurred in the past decades is the advent of colored elastic ties that hold the wires to the braces. Kids—and even adults—love matching their wires to their school colors, or favorite sports team, or even dance dress. They can change the color each time they change the wires, so it never gets old. It's always struck me as amusing that some patients, while still worrying about having braces and them being too noticeable, will then pick colors to make them even more obvious.

Technology has also reduced the amount of time you need to be in braces. Of course, it all depends on the difficulty of the problem, but in general, processes such as SureSmile have reduced the average length of treatment by almost one-third. In my office, during my first twenty years of treating about twelve thousand patients, the average time in braces was around twenty-three months. Since we adopted SureSmile in the late 2000s, our average time in braces has dropped to under sixteen months. Less complicated cases can often be done in less than a year.

SURESMILE

One of the ways innovative advances have impacted orthodontics is to take standard processes or hardware and make the ordinary extraordinary. The SureSmile process is a great example. SureSmile was developed in the mid-2000s by combining the emerging fields of 3-D imaging, digital manipulation of these images, and robotics.

I have been treating patients with the SureSmile system since 2007 and have completed treatment on more than thirty-five hundred patients using SureSmile. As far as I'm concerned, it's the best, most accurate, and fastest way to get your teeth straight. I'd been using conventional braces and wires for twenty years—and they did a great job and many, many patients were transformed by great smiles. But when something better comes along, I'd be doing a disservice to my patients not to jump at the chance to adopt it.

From the patient's point of view, the technology doesn't seem that revolutionary. We use exactly the same brackets that we use for any standard application—metal, clear ceramic, or lingual. The bracket is of no consequence. And nothing in the application process is different. What *is* different are the special prescription wires and the sophisticated way we develop a treatment plan for these patients.

First, SureSmile allows for a detailed 3-D treatment planning process, so instead of using 2-D x-rays and static plaster models, the patient's teeth, roots, and bone can be manipulated in a virtual 3-D environment. Second, the

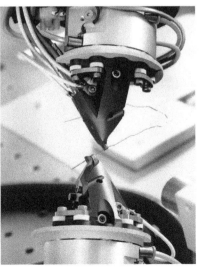

SureSmile wire-bending robot.

actual movements of the teeth are calculated to the nearest 0.1 mm. Third, the teeth are moved into their final positions with super-accurate, super-elastic, wires that are bent by a robot, instead of by hand. Yes, I'm afraid robots can do a better job making cars and TVs, vacuuming your carpet, and bending super-elastic orthodontic wires. Not even the most

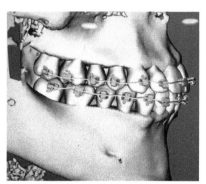

SureSmile scan image of teeth, bone, braces, and wire.

highly skilled orthodontist can bend a wire to within the accuracy of 0.1 millimeter.

When using SureSmile, we start off putting the braces on the teeth just like we did for patients for before we started using SureSmile. Then, usually two to eight months later, after some initial movement of teeth has taken place and some bite correction has been made, we do a 3-D scan of the teeth and the braces. The 3-D scan produces a digital, 3-D, CAD/CAM-like model of the teeth. The beauty of the 3-D scan is not only do we see the teeth, but we also see the roots and the bones that support the teeth.

Once we have that scan, I can go on my computer and perfect the treatment plan. I can move the teeth on the computer screen until the patient has a great smile and bite. I look at multiple views and make multiple tweaks until I get everything perfect. The SureSmile software allows for the soft tissue (lips, chin, nose) to be projected onto the teeth and bone. Remember, orthodontics is more than just straight teeth. It's a balance of teeth, bite, lips, smile line, and facial aesthetics. SureSmile really enhances this process.

Once I'm satisfied, I upload the digital file to the SureSmile digital lab, and robots go to work to provide a series of precisely bent wires that gently move the teeth into position. As I stated above, the robots do a much better job bending the wire than an orthodontist can do by hand. In addition, the wire is made of a special alloy that produces a gentle, constant force without losing its shape. This has been shown to be the best and most accurate way to move teeth with less discomfort than standard wires. Because the wires are bent by robotics, the pressure is just right—not too strong, not too soft.

With all this technology, patients don't feel or see anything different, but they definitely appreciate the shorter treatment time. Because SureSmile wires are so precise and efficient, we can usually reduce treatment time from about twenty-four months to about sixteen months, or even shorter for less-difficult problems. In addition, because the wires hold their ability to exert pressure longer than conventional wires, we can spread out appointments, so instead of coming in every four weeks, patients only come back every six to eight weeks. The overall shorter treatment time and the fewer appointments needed to carry out the treatment plan means patients and their parents are spending less of their time and effort on braces than ever before.

CLEAR ALIGNERS

Clear aligners have been the most significant addition to a patient's treatment options since I became an orthodontist thirty years ago. You only have to look at the exponential jump in adult patients to see the impact they have had.

Invisalign is, of course, the most well-known type. Its name has almost become synonymous with clear aligners, the way Kleenex now means any tissue and Googling refers to looking for information on any web browser. Whether Invisalign or another system, these aligners all function in a similar way. We offer both Invisalign, as well as SureClear aligners, which are manufactured by the same company that provides us with the prescription, robotically bent wire for braces.

How do clear aligners work?

No matter which system you use, as stated above, they move the teeth in a similar way. To move a tooth, you have to apply some force or pressure to the tooth. With braces, this is the wire, rubber bands, little springs, and various other "appliances." With clear aligners, it is the difference in the shape of one aligner compared to the next one that moves the tooth. For most patients, you'll have a series of upper and lower aligners (though sometimes we'll do braces on either the top or bottom and clear aligners in the other arch). The number of aligners needed to finish treatment successfully mainly depends on the complexity of the problem. Each aligner is manufactured to fit snugly and exert constant pressure on the teeth to move them into place. The patient changes to new aligners every one to two weeks, depending on the case.

The process of fitting the aligners and designing a treatment plan begins with either a 3-D scan or dental impressions. If your clear aligner dentist or orthodontist is still using dental impressions for Invisalign, I'd seriously question how up-to-date they are. 3-D scans provide much more accurate representations of the teeth than do old fashioned impressions, plus they are a heck of a lot easier on you, the patient.

In our office, the a 3-D scanner produces a 3-D image of the teeth. These scans are digitally transferred to a central lab, where 3-D virtual models are created from which a detailed treatment plan can be formulated. The treatment plan is created based on how, where, and when I want to move certain teeth. Many dentists and some orthodontists, who are not as experienced in Invisalign, will usually rely on the lab to interpret the scans and determine a plan. But I've been doing this long enough that I know what adjustments and tweaks should be made for the perfect smile—and there are always adjustments and tweaks.

For clear aligners, you often have to place "attachments" on the teeth, so the plastic can grab onto the more-rounded types of teeth. These attachments are little drops or little squares of that same composite material that we use to glue the braces on. Without these attachments, the aligners would fail to work or the treatment time would be very slow. How many teeth need attachments depends on the type of movement I'm looking for.

The clear aligner treatment is incremental. The patient wears each aligner somewhere between one and two weeks, and then changes the aligner to the next one in the series. Each aligner is shaped a little bit differently. So, it's that pressure of the plastic and the difference in the shape of the aligner that slowly move the teeth. To keep that pressure on, patients wear the aligners at least twenty-two hours a day. Most people snap them in and don't even know they are there. They fit so snuggly that you can do almost any activity with them, including sports, speaking, and playing musical instruments.

How many aligners will I need and does the treatment take longer than braces?

How many aligners you need and how often you'll change them depends on the problem we are correcting. For example, closing extra space between teeth usually take less time than the opposite problem of crowded teeth. The time for the overall treatment for braces and aligners is usually very similar, with some exceptions. One cool thing about aligner treatment is the software prediction outcomes, which give an accurate estimate of overall treatment time. You will be shown this software prediction the day your first aligners are placed.

What are the advantages and disadvantages of clear aligners?

The advantages of clear aligners are pretty obvious. They are practically invisible, so they are a good choice for adults and teens who feel braces are not for them. They usually require fewer office visits because the patient is given anywhere from five to eight aligners at a time and only needs to return to the office for the next check-up and to be given the next series of aligners. Another advantage is there are rarely any emergency visits. There are no wires to poke or braces to come loose. The other great advantage of clear aligners is being able to remove them for eating and brushing. You can eat whatever you want without having to cut it up or otherwise change your eating habits. One thing you must avoid, just like with braces, is sugary and acidic drinks. Of course, brushing and, in particular, flossing is much easier than with braces. And no one needs to worry that they have spinach stuck in a bracket during a business meeting!

The primary disadvantage of clear aligner treatment is that the patient must be responsible and, above all, consistent in wearing the aligners. The aligners need to be cleaned every day. They need to be taken out to eat. They need to be removed if you drink anything other than water. You need to brush your teeth well before putting them back in. If you're the type of person who doesn't think they are able to consistently wear the aligners—and a lot people, if they are honest with themselves, know this would be hard for them because they are too busy or eat too often (i.e., growing teenage boys) or are speaking all the time and worry the aligners will affect their speech—then clear aligners probably aren't for you. Just like the headgear of yesterday, it's all patient dependent. If you don't wear them that ideal twenty-two hours a day, they're not going to work.

Invisalign and SureSmile aligners have a lot of advantages, but you need to know that it's not a passive process. That all being said, the vast majority of patients, including most teenagers, do very well with clear aligners and are treated successfully.

Invisalign and SureSmile aligners have a lot of advantages, but you need to know that it's not a passive process.

One final disadvantage of Invisalign, SureSmile aligners and other clear aligner systems is that there are just some problems that are too difficult or challenging to treat with clear aligners. The expertise of a board-certified orthodontist, who has treated hundreds of patients with Invisalign, is invaluable. I have had to re-treat more than a handful of patients treated with Invisalign by less-experienced practitioners. Did you know that to become a "certified Invisalign provider" you only need to attend a two-day weekend course? Sometimes, the lack of a good outcome was because the provider didn't understand how the teeth moved with clear aligners. Other times, these were cases that were just far too difficult and involved to treat with clear aligners. In the latter types of cases, I converted them to braces, and they were finished successfully. In some particular patients, there may be one or two teeth that can't be moved very well with aligners. In these cases, we can put some partial braces on a few teeth to correct that specific problem and then convert to clear aligners for the rest of the treatment.

At-home orthodontics

A very recent phenomenon is a kind of do-it-yourself, at-home clear aligner program. At the time of this book's publication, the most familiar is "Smile Direct Club." Smile Direct Club advertises itself as an easy, low-cost, no appointment alternative to seeing an orthodontist or dentist for your clear aligner treatment. You take an impression of your teeth yourself with a kit they send you (good luck with that) or in some larger communities there are storefront scanning centers next to your local Starbucks. You never actually see or are evaluated by a trained dentist, let alone an orthodontist. Your case is "approved" or "rejected" remotely, and aligners shipped to your home. You wear and change the aligners as you do with Invisalign. The problem is most patients who "qualify" for Smile Direct Club involve crowding of the lower front teeth, and often there isn't room to move them because of the bite. The teeth can be straightened but the bite is messed up—then who do you turn to for correction? The barista at Starbucks? They also exaggerate the cost saving. Simple orthodontic cases that can be treated at home with Smile Direct Club are much less expensive in my office than a full set of braces or Invisalign. Buyer beware of DIY orthodontics.

LINGUAL BRACKETS

Lingual braces are small, metal brackets glued to the back of the teeth. The primary advantage is that they aren't seen at all. This is a huge advantage for some people. Lingual braces are great for those patients who, for whatever reason, don't want to show braces but are too difficult

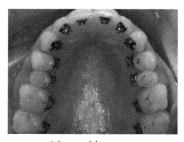

Lingual braces.

to treat with Invisalign or who have decided that wearing aligners consistently would be difficult.

The primary disadvantage to lingual braces is that there's a longer period of adjustment getting used to them. For some reason, the cheeks and the lips seem to adapt within a few days to braces on the outside of the teeth, whereas the tongue can take a week or so to get used to lingual braces. For this reason, as well as the fact it's just harder to work on the backside of the teeth than on the front, we rarely use lingual braces on the bottom teeth. We usually put lingual braces just on the top teeth and clear ceramic brackets or clear aligners on the lower teeth.

Treatment can take a little bit longer with lingual braces, just because of the shape of the wires and the mechanics of the system. However, with lingual braces, we always use the SureSmile system of 3-D imaging and prescription robotically bent wires. This has greatly increased the efficiency of lingual braces reducing overall treatment time.

CERAMIC BRACKETS

Ceramic brackets are clear or tooth-colored brackets, made from ceramic (hence the name), porcelain, or, sometimes, plastic. In my office, we use ceramic-based brackets because we trust their durability. They are similar to metal brackets. They go on the teeth the same way. They stay on the teeth the same way. You will have the same number of appointments and the same length of treatment as you would with traditional metal brackets. The only difference is that some ceramic brackets are a bit larger. Because the material is just a bit more brittle than metal, they need to be slightly larger to be strong enough to handle the wire. Although ceramic isn't quite as strong as metal, some people think the brackets have a habit of breaking. This is a false assumption. While the material itself might not be as strong, the manufacturing process accounts for that, so the final ceramic bracket is no more likely to break or come loose than a metal bracket.

The advantage of ceramic brackets is that they are less noticeable. Because they are clear or tooth-colored, your eye doesn't immediately jump to them when someone opens their mouth.

The only downside to ceramic brackets is the larger size. The smaller metal brackets are easier to clean around, and thus hygiene is easier. Also, some people with particularly sensitive mouths have trouble getting used to them. In these cases, we might use ceramic just on the front top teeth, and traditional metal braces on the other, less-seen teeth.

For someone who wants or needs traditional braces to straighten their teeth but doesn't want to flash metal every time they smile, ceramic brackets are a good compromise.

MIXING AND MATCHING

Each treatment option has its own advantages and disadvantages. Sometimes, however, the best treatment plan is combination therapy, which involves more than one option. For example, the patient might have a minor problem with their top teeth and more severe crowding on the bottom. In this type of case, we can use clear aligners for the top teeth, and regular braces on the bottom. Since most people don't show the lower teeth as much, they are more apt to accept that type of combination treatment.

Sometimes, a patient really wants to have Invisalign, but they have one or two teeth that are rotated or otherwise significantly out of alignment. Invisalign doesn't handle those types of situations very well. To rectify this problem, we can place three or four braces just in one area of the mouth for three or four months to get that one tooth where we need it to be. And then we can transition to Invisalign.

Orthodontics is no longer a one-size-fits-all proposition. In my office, innovative technology and a variety of options result in very individualized treatment plans. Patients can be confident that they will walk out with a smile that fits their face—and spend very little time getting there.

LOOKING TO THE FUTURE

Because braces are so ubiquitous, researchers are doubling down in trying to find ways to make treatment plans more efficient and more comfortable. Patients are simply demanding better experiences and orthodontists are working to provide that.

One of the more interesting areas of research is looking at why Johnny's teeth move faster than Joey's teeth. Is there a genetic component? Is there a pill Joey can take or a compound we can put on his teeth or a treatment we can offer to make Joey's teeth move as easily as Johnny's? There is nothing on the horizon yet, but researchers are diving deep into the physiology. If we could crack that puzzle, orthodontics would take a giant leap forward.

There are also some devices that supposedly increase the speed of which teeth move. One of them looks like a vibrating mouth guard that is supposed to increase blood flow to the tooth root and gums, and thus increase the rate of movement. Recent research seems to indicate that it doesn't really work, but it's an intriguing idea. Another device uses pulsating ultraviolet light, but again, clinical research has yet to determine if it makes teeth move faster. The holy grail is to find a way to move teeth faster and easier. Each innovation brings us closer.

CHAPTER 6

Getting from Here to There

*Smile. It instantly lifts the face
and just lights up the room.*
CHRISTIE BRINKLEY

I n this chapter, I'm going to walk you through what happens when you come in the first time for a consultation all the way through to completing your treatment with braces or clear aligners. No matter what option you choose, the process is relatively the same— friendly, patient focused, and straightforward.

CHOOSING AN ORTHODONTIST

Most of my patients find us in one of three ways. First of all, about one-third of our patients come from their dentist sending them directly to our office. However, unlike many medical insurance plans, no one needs a referral from their family dentist to see an orthodontist. However, because dentists are often your primary contact, it's very common for your dentist to be the first one to notice that your teeth are misaligned, or that your bite is off. Most dentists have a couple of orthodontists in their communities that they are comfortable recommending to patients.

Maybe a few more than one-third come to us via word of mouth. One mom talks to another at the soccer game or the grocery story. One kid likes the colored braces on a friend's teeth and asks who their orthodontist is. With so many kids in braces during middle school, it's not hard for a parent looking for a recommendation to simply turn to the parent sitting next to them at back-to-school night. And, of course, many of my current patients had older siblings whom we treated. Adult patients often begin treatment after they see the difference it has made in their children's lives.

The rest come to us after doing an internet search. This is becoming much more common and has increased dramatically in the past few years. In fact, I wouldn't be surprised if I took a formal poll of my patients to find that this group is bigger than I think. Whether it's social media posts, Google or Yelp reviews, or my practice's or personal Facebook pages, more and more people are looking to the web in researching their orthodontic treatment. Reading Internet reviews on an orthodontic practice has become today's parents' "word of mouth."

No matter how they come to us, patients generally want to know four things before they proceed with treatment: What's wrong? What do I need to do to correct it? How long is it going to take? How much is it going to cost?

Once we are able to answer those questions—and we always do—we are ready to get at it.

THAT FIRST APPOINTMENT

Meeting new patients is my absolute favorite thing to do as an orthodontist. I meet so many wonderful people and try to set their minds at ease about orthodontic treatment. My staff and I see our roles as educational. It is extremely easy to schedule that first appointment. Simply call the office. We like to personally talk to the parent or patient to make sure we have answered all

Meeting new patients is my absolute favorite thing to do as an orthodontist.

of their questions and that they feel comfortable with our process. You'll also be sent a secure link to forward personal, health, and insurance information to our office at your convenience.

Like most orthodontists today, we do not charge for the initial consultation visit, and neither do we bill any insurance you may have until actual treatment has begun. This is why we encourage families to have all children seven years or older screened, and we like to schedule multiple family members together. The first appointment is a one-hour consultation. During this first visit, you'll work with a Treatment Coordinator. My Treatment Coordinators are our knowledgeable staff members who will guide you through the new patient process.

We take pictures and scans

First of all, we take photographs of the face and smile, as well as a series of digital photographs of your teeth and bite.

We'll also obtain a 3-D cone beam image. The scanner rotates around the patient, capturing data using a cone-shaped, low-dose x-ray beam. The resulting images are used to construct a 3-D image of the patient's teeth, mouth, and jaw. Some patients worry about the radiation exposure, but it is a really negligible dose. We have the latest 3-D system, and the exposure to x-rays from this scan is about the same as the old x-rays dentists took between the teeth. It's so much less than you would be exposed to from a medical or hospital CT scan.

I'll do an examination

Next, I'll do an examination and take specific measurements. In the vast majority of cases, based on my thirty-plus years of experience treating more than twenty thousand patients, I can formulate a detailed treatment action plan during this first visit. I'll tweak the actual measurements and treatment plan using modeling software, but I usually know what the approach will be. For that remaining 5 percent or so, I may have to do some further analysis or perhaps contact an orthodontic colleague about the treatment. In those more difficult cases, we would have the patient and their family back for a second visit to formalize the treatment options.

We present a treatment plan

We then spend time going over our proposed plan with the parent or patient. Typically, the goal is the same for most patients: Straight teeth, great smile aesthetics, a good bite, and optimal positioning of the teeth in the bone for long-term dental health. Though the treatment objectives are universal, as we stated in the previous chapter, there may be several ways to achieve the finished treatment. We'll cover all the options: braces, SureSmile, clear aligners, and combination treatment, and I'll let you know which method or methods best suits your particular case.

The goal can be a little different with adults. With children, because they will be living with their teeth for seventy or eighty years, we strive for an ideal result—the ideal smile, the ideal bite—even if some of the things we correct aren't obvious to an outside observer. To get this ideal outcome, it may require more work or more expense than some adults want to put into it. In those cases, we would just give them an aesthetic option. Instead of trying to correct everything, they just want to have a nicer smile, a nicer appearance. That's an option for adults, who make their own decisions.

When we are presenting the treatment plan, we put everything on a large flat screen monitor and walk the patient through the process step by step. "We have problem A, B, and C. This is the solution." First you describe the problem, and then you talk about the solutions to those problems. We also have a lot of video aides to explain the different appliances or different techniques that we use.

IT'S WORTH IT (HOW MUCH DOES THIS COST?)

"How much will it all cost?" is probably the one question everyone wants to ask right at the beginning, but often feel embarrassed to ask. They don't want to put a price on their child's health and happiness— or their own.

I would never tell someone that orthodontics is cheap. It's not. But the cost isn't outlandish, either, and it's well worth the investment. This isn't a one-time trip to a foreign city or a new car that will need to be replaced in a few years. This is an investment in your or

> **This is an investment in your or your child's future that will still be paying dividends fifty years from now, when they still have all their own teeth—and a great smile.**

your child's future that will still be paying dividends fifty years from now, when they still have all their own teeth—and a great smile. Remember the story back in Chapter 1 about the dad re-enforcing my message to his son about how his new smile was an investment and how he judged prospect employees by their smile?

Now, for many patients who need full comprehensive SureSmile braces or clear aligner treatment, it is probably wise to budget $5,000 to $6,000. Lingual braces and more-complicated cases will add to that fee. The cost of the orthodontic treatment depends on the length of time the treatment takes, and this depends on the issues being treated—it only makes sense that a more difficult, time-consuming treatment lasting a couple years will be costlier than a simple case taking a few months. Because cost is tied to the amount of time needed to get that perfect smile, less-complicated treatment plans will cost much less than more complicated plans. This is why we never estimate the cost of treatment without seeing the patient. We want to give accurate information based on a patient's individual needs.

We work with patients to find the best way to pay for the treatment because we do understand orthodontic treatment needs to be budgeted into the family's expenses. Many patients have insurance that covers part of the treatment fee. We communicate with your insurance company to find out exactly what is covered, and then we file claims for patients to make it easier for them to use their insurance. Others have Flexible Savings Accounts that can be used to offset the cost. For everyone, we can set up a payment plan with flexible down payment options and then monthly payments that stretch over the course of the treatment. It is rare in our office for my Treatment Coordinators to be unable to come up with a payment scenario that fits a family's budget.

GETTING STARTED

Once we've agreed on a treatment plan and how we are going to accomplish those treatment goals, and comfortable payment arrangements have been finalized, we are ready to start. Patients have the option of getting started right then and there or making another appointment and coming back to have the braces put on or start their clear aligner scans. Most are happy to have one less appointment and so they stay for the extra forty to fifty minutes it takes to apply brackets or do a 3-D scan for clear aligners.

If a patient has decided on clear aligners, we start by first polishing the teeth and then doing an intraoral scan. The technology of the scanners has improved greatly, and scans that used to take twenty to thirty minutes now take ten to fifteen. I assume that time will continue to decrease. We use both Invisalign and SureSmile aligners in our office, and the scanning process for the patient is the same for each. Once the scan is completed, the patient is done for the moment. It's fast and streamlined.

That 3-D scan is then transmitted to the clear aligner design company and converted into virtual 3-D patient models, from which a detailed treatment plan and aligner sequence can be formulated and adjusted to meet my exact treatment goals. Once the treatment plan is finalized, the aligners can be manufactured. We allow four weeks between the time of the clear aligner scan to when the aligners are delivered to the patient.

At the delivery appointment, we again polish the teeth and then place the small attachments on the teeth that need them. Placing the attachment is similar to the process of gluing braces on but takes less time. The teeth are dried and isolated and the attachment placed in a matter of minutes. Then it is time to place and deliver the aligners. Our patient managers work with you on how to place and remove the aligners and go over all necessary care instructions. The coolest part of the first appointment is showing the patient the software prediction of how their teeth are going to move. How they are going to go from misaligned to beautiful.

Now, for braces with the SureSmile process, the sequence is kind of reversed. I apply the braces first, and then we do the SureSmile scan a bit later in the treatment. For most patients, we place both upper and lower braces at the first appointment. This take about forty to fifty minutes. For some patients, we only place the upper braces at the first appointment. This is usually done for two reasons: 1) The upper teeth overlap the lower front teeth too much to comfortably place the lower braces, and 2) There are impacted teeth in the upper arch and since this take time to correct, we delay placing lower braces until needed.

When we are ready to place the brackets. Teeth are dried and isolated. The braces are placed, and the adhesive is dried with an LED light. We then thread the first wires through the brackets, and you are on your way. Even if the patient has opted in to the SureSmile system, we start with our own wires, so the patient doesn't have to wait for the prescription wires to be molded and sent to the office. It's better to begin right away with a standard wire rather than wait several weeks. Remember, moving the teeth is a physiological process. So, you have to get the cells that make new bone and move the teeth activated. They have to get revved up. That's what the initial wire does. The scan for the SureSmile wires are done at a later appointment once the teeth have aligned somewhat.

After the braces are all attached, we spend quite a bit of time explaining how to care for them. In fact, I've included an entire chapter, so I won't go into detail here. But briefly—brush, brush, brush. Good hygiene is crucial. Without it, you can end up with damaged teeth and gums. That's not the outcome we want, particularly when it is easily preventable.

WORKING WITH THE FRONT DESK

When it's time to leave, the patient goes out to the front desk, where my team works with them to set up convenient follow-up appointments. The average time between appointments ranges from four to ten weeks, but six to seven weeks is average. Sometimes with clear aligners, it can even be a little bit longer, more like eight to ten weeks.

In any case, the follow-up appointment at four-week intervals are pretty much a thing of the past. Most of these adjustment appointments will take between twenty and thirty minutes. They can be as short as ten to fifteen minutes for simple wire checks or clear aligner changes.

We will also find out how you want to be contacted if we need to get in touch. After every appointment, I do a personal recap. If the parents are there, it is easy to talk right in the office. But if someone else has brought the child in, such as a grandparent or babysitter, we need to know how to get that recap to the parent. Because of privacy laws, we can't give it to the friendly neighbor who brought your child to our office when the parent couldn't. In most cases nowadays, parents like to be texted. We also do a lot of emails. However, people are getting less and less concerned about checking emails. So, we've found that texting is the best way to communicate.

The updates can be brief— "We saw Johnny today. We changed a wire and started him wearing rubber bands. Please make an appointment to follow up in seven weeks" —so texts are perfect.

THE FINAL APPOINTMENT

When treatment is done, removing the wire and brackets is done quickly and painlessly—usually in about two minutes. Then the adhesive is removed and the teeth are polished. This is the best day for everyone. Patients sometimes have a hard time sitting still because they are so excited. And I never get over the feeling that I've really helped someone, maybe even changed their entire life.

> I never get over the feeling that I've really helped someone, maybe even changed their entire life.

We usually place the retainers a day or two after the braces have been removed. For clear aligner patients, their retainers can be placed the same day as we remove the attachments.

Next to seeing new patients, this is my favorite appointment, when we look at the before-and-after photographs with the patients and their families and ask if their friends or colleagues have noticed their great new smile. We fit the patient for retainers that we hope they will wear for many years and go over care instructions, just like we did when they were first fitted with aligners or braces. Retainers are extremely important. No matter how great the outcome at the time braces are removed, teeth have a tendency to move if not held in place with a retainer. For some patients, that movement will never be noticeable. For others, by the time they are in their thirties or forties, they will be coming back for a tune up. Ideally, we recommend long-term retainer wear. I always tell patients. "You should wear your retainers as long as you want your teeth to stay straight."

The primary problem with wearing retainers is actually wearing them. We suggest that patients keep their retainers next to their bed or near their toothbrush, so they don't forget each night. Just make sure the dog can't get it. For some reason, dogs love to chew up retainers.

I fortunately now have 3-D printing, so we give each patient two sets of retainers and the 3-D printed models they were made from. With these 3-D printed models, it's easy to create a replacement retainer as long as your teeth have not shifted. All you have to do is call. And if you have an interesting story of how you lost all of them, we'd love to hear it.

Although getting your braces removed and placing retainers is technically the end of your treatment, we are always available to answer questions or to schedule a quick follow up appointment if you have concerns. Straight teeth should be that way for a lifetime, and we're there to make sure they stay that way.

CHAPTER 7

Life with Braces

*A smile is the light in your window
that tells others that there is a caring
sharing person inside.*
DENNIS WAITLEY

Now that you have your braces or clear aligners, you need to know how to take care of them. Patients often wonder if there will be any restrictions on food, drink, or activities. The easy answer is, "There should be no restrictions on activities, but you will want to be careful with what you eat." The more nuanced answers are outlined in the rest of the chapter.

THOSE FIRST FEW DAYS

During the first couple of days with braces, your cheeks and lips will be getting used to the wires and brackets. Typically, by the end of the third day, you won't even notice that you have braces. If you have lingual braces, it will take your tongue a little longer to adapt than it takes cheeks and lips, but it will soon adapt, as well.

Clear aligners can take up to a week for your mouth to get to the point that it stops sending signals to your brain to "get these things out!" The aligners are larger than metal brackets. They cover the entire tooth, including a little bit of the gums, so there is just more to get used to. But your lips, cheeks, and gums will soon get used to the aligners, and you won't notice them at all.

Some patients also report that they have a hard time speaking clearly. This comes up more with lingual braces and aligners than with standard braces. But this, too, shall pass. Your tongue and lips will adjust in just a few days, and no one will be able to tell from your speech that you have braces.

There is no one-size-fits-all for how patients adjust to having brackets, wires, or aligners in their mouth.

There is no one-size-fits-all for how patients adjust to having brackets, wires, or aligners in their mouth. The vast majority are simply aware that they have something on their teeth for a couple of days, and then don't feel anything. If, however, the brackets or wires are irritating or rubbing against your cheeks or lips, we give you some wax to place on the brackets to soften their edges. Just ask someone in the office, and they will be happy to provide it. Your cheeks will get used to the brackets, and you'll only need the wax for a couple of days.

Your gums and teeth may be sore and tender beginning the second day and continuing for a day or two more. We are moving your teeth, after all. It's more of an achy feeling than real pain; it's not a sharp pain but just a dull ache. For many patients, it's not a big deal. They aren't bothered enough to do anything about it. Others find that dissolving a teaspoon of salt in a cup of lukewarm water and swishing the solution in their mouth for just a couple of minutes is soothing (do not swallow the salt water). Still others prefer to take over-the-counter pain relievers until the achiness passes. Know that whether the soreness is extremely minor or irritating enough to take ibuprofen, it will be gone within a few days.

Patients often have the misconception that aligners will not cause the same soreness as braces. This is a very false assumption. The teeth don't know whether braces and wires are moving them, or that aligners are moving them. So, with aligners, you get soreness, too. In fact, you might experience more days of mild soreness because we are changing the aligners every week or two rather than changing wires every six weeks, the way we do with standard braces. Every time you put that new aligner in, you're going to have a little soreness for a day or two. If you have aligners, you need to make sure that you leave them in, even if your teeth are sore.

After about a week, most patients are through that initial period, and most won't even remember they have braces unless they are looking in a mirror.

One thing that sometimes panics patients is the feeling that one or more of their teeth feel loose. This isn't common, but it's not rare either. If you feel this sensation, don't worry. Your teeth are moving, and the tooth socket is getting slightly larger, so teeth can feel a little mobile. It will soon tighten up and feel just as attached as it always has.

EATING WITH BRACES

Eating with braces is an adjustment, but it's not difficult. It's more simply being aware of what you are eating and the impact it might have on your braces. During the first few days, you are going to want to stick to soft foods, not only because the adhesive that holds the brackets on the teeth is still setting up, but just to give yourself a day or two to get used to the feel of the braces. Chewing and swallowing will have a slightly different feel with the brackets and wires on.

The first day or two, we recommend a very soft diet—yogurt,

well-cooked pasta, mashed potatoes, soups, things like that. You want to avoid trying to bite into anything until the second or third day. When you do bite into food, you have to be a bit more careful. You can't, for example, bite into an apple. You have to cut the apple up and chew it. You can't rip a piece of pizza off with your front teeth. You certainly don't want to chew hard or sticky candy that might stick to your teeth or pull the braces off.

Foods that are best to avoid tend to be sticky foods, such as caramel and chewy candy; crunchy foods, such as popcorn and ice; and hard foods, such as nuts and bread sticks. Most patients intuitively know to avoid sticky and hard foods. What they often don't realize, however, is the effect sugary and acidic foods can have on their teeth when they wear braces. A diet high in sugar can cause the area around the bracket to decalcify, leaving a little white square on the teeth when the braces are removed. One of the saddest things we see is when we take the braces off and there's a little white square left on the tooth around where the bracket was glued on. This decalcification is caused by a combination of poor oral hygiene and, more importantly, high sugar content in the diet. In fact, patients that actually have pretty good brushing habits can still get this decalcification if they have a lot of sugar in the diet.

Avoiding high-sugar foods is really important when you have braces on. Obviously, there are some foods that are no-brainers when it comes to identifying them as having a high sugar content—candies, ice cream, bakery goods, etc. But there's a lot of hidden sugars in our foods, as well. Sports drinks have a lot of sugar. Fruit juices have a lot of sugar. It doesn't matter if it's natural or processed, sugar is sugar. If you're the type of patient that sips on sports drinks, soft drinks, or sugar-loaded coffee all day, and doesn't brush after each drink is done, you're really susceptible to this decalcification. We also see this type of decalcification in people who suck on mints.

We really try to keep an eye on that. This is a permanent blemish on the tooth, so we want to avoid it at all cost. As soon as we notice it, we alert the patient and ask them to examine their diet and eliminate the sources of sugar that are affecting their teeth.

Conversely, and this doesn't happen nearly as often as people taking in too much sugar, is having too many acidic foods in your diet. For example, if you're sucking on lemons with braces on, you could end up with a situation similar to decalcification where what was healthy enamel around the braces is eaten away by the acidic foods.

When we talk to our patients about foods to avoid, they always ask about gum. Everyone assumes that gum is off the table. To their surprise, we actually encourage them to chew sugarless gum. If you chew sugar-free gum, it increases the saliva in the mouth, which decreases things like cavities and decalcification. It's perfectly fine to chew sugarless gum with braces on. Just be sure that's what you're chewing. You don't want to accidentally buy regular gum, which not only contains too much sugar, but is much stickier and, thus, harder on your braces.

You can eat most foods. You just have to modify how you do it and how you chew. Patients are always a little hesitant about biting things in the beginning, but as you get used to the braces, you just become more and more comfortable chewing and knowing what you can eat and what you cannot eat.

One of the main advantages of Invisalign and other clear aligners is that you don't need to worry about what you eat. Because you remove the aligners when you eat, there is no danger that they will be damaged by chewing. Even if you want to, it's almost impossible to eat with aligners on—you end up just mashing the food rather than biting or chewing it. I've tried it and its not any fun. Of course, we recommend that whenever possible that you brush your teeth after eating and before you put the aligners back in. But be careful with them; more than one patient has called to tell us that they've left the aligners in a restaurant or on a plane or at their grandparents' house or accidently threw them away. You do still need to watch your sugar and acid intake. Now those attachments used to help anchor the aligners act the same way as brackets when exposed to too much sugar or acid. So, you really have to avoid sugary drinks and sugar when you have the aligners. Patients can drink with the aligners in their mouth, but they should be aware of the sugar content of those drinks. For example, there is a lot of sugar in some coffee drinks. If you do drink something sugary and you have your aligners in, then you want to try to rinse out with water as soon as you can.

LOOSE WIRES AND BRACKETS

The wires and brackets on your braces are really strong, but they can break or come loose. If this happens, simply call the office and we'll get you in to fix the problem. If you like do-it-yourself projects, you can often temporarily fix loose wires by using the eraser end of pencil (not the other end) or other non-pointy object to gently push the wire back into the bracket. If the loose wire is causing irritation to your lips or cheeks, you can put wax or a wet cotton ball over the broken wire to relieve the pain until we can get it repaired.

About 5 percent of the braces come loose at some point, so it's not a major tragedy if you have a brace come loose. It becomes a major issue if it happens so often that it interferes with the treatment plan. If a bracket is off a tooth, or a wire has pulled loose, then that tooth or section of teeth isn't getting the consistent pressure it needs to move into place. If a brace isn't on the tooth, that tooth isn't moving.

If this is happening a lot, you need to look at what you are eating.

These brackets generally don't jump off by themselves while you are sleeping. It is almost always related to doing something you really shouldn't be—chewing ice or nuts, eating caramels, absentmindedly picking at a bracket with a pen while studying.

PLAYING SPORTS AND INSTRUMENTS WITH BRACES

Many new patient ask if they can still play sports with braces on. Of course, you can! We only ask that all athletes wear a mouth guard to protect their teeth and braces. In fact, we'd recommend mouth guards for all athletes, whether they wear braces or not. Why wouldn't you want to protect your teeth?

We only ask that all athletes wear a mouth guard to protect their teeth and braces. In fact, we'd recommend mouth guards for all athletes, whether they wear braces or not.

So, we encourage mouth guards on all our patients for almost every sport. Many sports require mouth guards—football, hockey, lacrosse, wrestling, to name a few. We have special mouth guards that fit over the braces that we give to these athletes at no charge. Soccer and basketball, on the other hand, often don't require mouth guards, which always baffles me. Neither do baseball or softball. Kids are running full speed into each other, elbows are flying, balls are being thrown and/or kicked. It just completely befuddles me that mouth guards aren't required. Whether required or not, we ask that our patients wear them. You don't want to destroy all that work your braces have been doing. If you're being treated with clear aligners, it is best to wear a sports mouth guard for contact sports, then place the aligners back in once your practice or game is over.

If your braces are damaged during a sports activity, all you have to do is call the office and we'll repair any damage. If your cheeks or lips have been injured, rinsing your mouth with salt water will clean any cuts, while soothing the damaged tissue.

We are also often asked about how braces or clear aligners will affect the patient's ability to continue to play their flute or trombone. The answer for aligners is easy: here is no impact. The patient simply removes the aligners while they are practicing or playing and carries on as normal. (Please put those aligners back in as soon as you are finished, to keep your treatment plan on track.)

How standard braces affect a patient's ability to play an instrument is more nuanced. It depends if it's a brass instrument, a flute or a piccolo, or a woodwind instrument. The easiest instruments to get used to are a clarinet or a saxophone, where the mouthpiece goes inside the mouth. Other instrument, such as a flute, where you are blowing over the instrument, or a brass instrument, such as a baritone, trumpet, or trombone, where the mouthpiece is placed in front of your teeth, will be harder to get used to. If you look at any middle school or high school marching band or orchestra, you will see as many kids in braces as you'll see in any gathering of young teens. It takes some practice and experimentation, but by the first adjustment appointment, all of our patients have figured out how to play their musical instruments.

CLEANING YOUR BRACES

Dental hygiene is very, very important when wearing braces. Food and plaque accumulate more easily around braces making you more susceptible to gingivitis, periodontal disease and cavities.

We often get asked if the patient should invest in an electric toothbrush or a water flosser or water pick to make sure all food is removed. While those devices can certainly help, the most important thing is to brush well and often, whether you're using a manual toothbrush or an electric toothbrush. You have to take the time to brush after every meal and take the time to do a good job while brushing. The biggest problem we have is with younger patients. Most adults are pretty good at it. When we see problems with hygiene, it's not because of the type of brush they are using; it's the lack of effort and attention to brush well.

All that being said, electric toothbrushes really does do a better job cleaning around the braces than a manual toothbrush does. Water picks will also help remove food particles between teeth. But patients can certainly get by with a manual toothbrush and flossing if they don't want to invest in an electric toothbrush and water pick.

As for flossing, this can be a definite challenge with braces. Superfloss, floss with a built-in threader, and small proxy brushes, are what we recommend in lieu of trying to manipulate the floss under the wires and between the teeth.

We've been focusing on dental hygiene for braces, but there are a few things you should know about clear aligners. First of all, aligners are much easier to keep clean than are braces. You take them out for eating, so you are able to continue to brush and floss just as you did before you got aligners. The main thing to remember is that you need to brush each time before putting the aligners back in. If you put the aligners in without brushing, you run the risk of trapping food (and sugar) between the aligner and the teeth. Not only does it look awful, but it also opens you up to cavities and gum disease.

BOTTOM LINE

So, bottom line for this chapter? Getting used to your braces and aligners will take a few days. However, as millions of patients have done before you and millions will afterwards, eating, brushing, and playing sports and musical instruments can readily be done with braces and clear aligners.

Finally, it is a requirement for our patients that they continue to see their family dentist and hygienist for scheduled check-ups and cleanings. If we see patients that are less than diligent with their oral hygiene, we'll recommend three-month dental cleanings rather than the normal six months.

CHAPTER 8

Clearing Up the Myths

Most smiles are started by another smile.

ANONYMOUS

O rthodontics is so common now that everyone thinks they know all about it and what you don't you can always find the most accurate information on the web, right? They know what they do, they know what they cost, they know what you can and can't do while wearing them. When questioned, however, it usually turns out people don't know as much as they think. There are a lot of myths out there that are so common that they're often just accepted as fact. I'd like to use this chapter to clear up some of the more common orthodontic myths. Some used to be thought to be true, but research has proven them false. And some were never true, but sound like they should be. Follow me, and I'll point you in the right direction. Please remember, everything you read in a Google search is not necessarily accurate; and that is true.

MYTH: You need a referral from the dentist to see an orthodontist.

REALITY: You do not need a referral from your dentist or anyone else to see an orthodontist for an evaluation.

Because most people now belong to medical insurance plans or groups that require a referral from their primary physician to visit a specialist, they think the same relationship exists between dentists and orthodontists. It doesn't. Dentists often *do* refer patients to me. Patients will arrive with a form that notes what the dentist saw and the suggestion to see me. But you don't need a referral to visit my practice, and neither do you have to go to the orthodontist that your dentist suggests. In fact, most of my patients come to me via word of mouth, as relatives of current patients or through an internet search. It's great if a dentist refers someone, and I appreciate that the dentist is providing the best service possible to their patients by letting them know when orthodontics would be helpful, but it's not a requirement for treatment.

MYTH: You don't need to see your regular dentist while in braces or clear aligners.

REALITY: You definitely do need to see your regular dentist at least every six months, or as often as you did before starting braces.

In fact, I'd say it's even more important to see your dentist for routine cleaning and gum inspections when you are in braces than when you aren't. While conscientious patients are great at keeping their teeth clean, nothing beats a professional cleaning at your dentist. You can brush after every meal, but your hygienist can see where you might be missing when cleaning those back teeth. Plus, he or she has specialized instruments to really get all the plaque and tartar off. Having braces makes your teeth a little more challenging to clean. Don't pass up the chance to have your regular dentist help out.

MYTH: **Braces are painful.**

REALITY: **Technology has come a long way in making braces more comfortable than ever before.**

There was a time, thirty years or so ago, when having braces put on was, indeed, painful. The bands that went around the teeth had to be pushed on up into the gum line, and this would hurt. Today, as mentioned in an earlier chapter, we painlessly glue brackets onto the front of the teeth. Teeth might be sore after each adjustment, but they are not painful in the sense that stubbing your toe is painful. You will probably experience just a mild achiness when you bite into something for a day or so after a new wire or aligner is placed. Everybody has a different tolerance, but as far as braces or clear aligners being painful, I would say that's a wildly exaggerated characterization of the sensation.

MYTH: **Children's jaws will grow enough to so that crowded teeth will straighten themselves out.**

REALITY: **Not usually.**

At around age eight, the part of the jaw that accommodates the teeth is actually done growing in width. Yes, the jaw grows, but only in length to make space for erupting twelve-year molars and eventually wisdom teeth.

MYTH: **If my child's teeth look straight, they don't need an orthodontic evaluation.**

REALITY: **Some orthodontic problems aren't visible to a parent or casual observer.**

There are a couple of special bite problems, where the teeth look good but the bite is way off. The most common is called a "deep bite," where the top teeth really overlap the bottom teeth, so you bite down hard on your bottom teeth. You can barely see the bottom teeth at all when you're biting down. Those types of patients are prone to severe wear of their lower incisor teeth; I've seen patients in their thirties and forties where those teeth are about half the size they should be. They've been worn down from natural chewing, because the bite is bad.

MYTH: **Removing teeth changes the look of your face.**
REALITY: **When done to mitigate severe overcrowding and when tooth movement is properly controlled there is little or no change to the facial profile.**

We don't often remove teeth any more—devices to expand the palate and give teeth more room have helped solve a lot of crowding problems—but there are still some situations where the teeth are so crowded the only solution is to remove a few to make room for those that remain. Patients sometimes worry that pulling those teeth will cause their lips to pull inward. They have visions of their grandparents without dentures. But this is not the case. The goal of orthodontics is to give you a great smile. We work with the jaw and lips to make sure we do. If you know how to control the movement of the teeth, like any good orthodontist should do, you're not going to see that deleterious change in the profile. Now, on the other hand, there are some situations where you want to change the profile. These are patients with crowding and teeth that protrude forward, making it difficult to close the lips. In these cases, we want to move the teeth inward and the lips also.

MYTH: **To get the best result, you have to wear headgear and other unflattering appliances.**
REALITY: **Not in my office or most orthodontist's now days.**

We don't use that. We've found we can fix the bite and realign the jaw using appliances that are in the mouth rather than around the head or neck.

MYTH: Invisalign or clear aligner treatment takes longer than braces.

REALITY: For most patients, this is not true.

As I stated earlier, the movement of teeth is a physiological process. Teeth and the surrounding bone don't know what is moving them. For most cases, the time to treat is very similar for clear aligners and braces. The biggest exception is patients that have deep bites, where the front teeth overlap and cover up the lower teeth. Correction of this does take longer with clear aligners.

MYTH: Everyone needs to have impressions of their mouths taken before they can get braces, and the material used to get impressions of your mouth tastes bad and often makes you gag.

REALITY: We rarely use impressions any more.

It's true that, in the past, we had to get impressions of everyone's mouth. How else were we going to know what the teeth and bite looked like? Back in those days, orthodontists often gave patients the molds of their before and after teeth as a souvenir. Today, we use 3-D scanners to get virtual pictures of your mouth. The molds used to be static, so you got what you got. Today's virtual scans can be manipulated so I can view the teeth and bite from a variety of angles, as well as move the teeth on screen to see how it will all end up. It's a much better process for both the patient and the orthodontist. When we do have to take impressions, the material is only in the mouth about thirty seconds though, instead of a couple minutes.

MYTH: All Invisalign (clear aligner) treatment is the same, so it doesn't matter if you use a dentist or an orthodontist or attempt an at home product.

REALITY: Experience and skill can make a tremendous difference in the final outcome of Invisalign treatment.

This myth is built on the fact that all Invisalign aligners come from a central lab. So, when an orthodontist or a dentist submits a case to Invisalign, the scans are all sent down to their lab in Costa Rica. We send along a checklist of how we want the teeth to move, and from there, it's taken over by a lab technician. They're not dentists or orthodontists. The plans are governed by the algorithms that Invisalign has developed that tells them, "If the scans show A, B, C, then we need to do this. If they show D, E, F, then we do something else."

So, unless you do a critical analysis of what you get back, you're just dependent on how the lab technician and the computer wants to move the teeth. Well, on a computer, you can move the teeth anywhere you want. It doesn't mean that's how they're going to move in a person's mouth, or how they're going to move in the bone.

Invisalign is a cookie-cutter process, unless you do a critical analysis of it, which we do with our all our cases. Whenever I get a case back from Invisalign, I usually have to send it back at least three or four times for them to make corrections and get it right. If you don't have that critical eye, you will just accept the plan and aligners that the lab technician sends back. That's how a lot of dentists and even some orthodontists use Invisalign, but it's not how we handle those cases in our office. We believe that interpreting the scans and plans makes a huge difference in the outcome for our patients.

MYTH: Clear aligners move the teeth differently than standard braces, so you don't need an orthodontist.

REALITY: A tooth doesn't know whether the force being applied is from plastic aligners or wires and brackets, so the underlying process is the same.

You still have to understand how the teeth move and in what direction, what magnitude you need to move a tooth, and when you should do it within the treatment timeline.

MYTH: Do-It-Yourself home programs are just as good as an orthodontist. And they are a lot cheaper!

REALITY: These programs can work in a limited number if the misalignment is minor and everything goes perfectly. But how often is everything perfect? Plus, they aren't cheaper than taking care of the same problem in an orthodontist's office.

Invisalign, the original clear aligner company, once had a monopoly on clear aligner products, however, many of their patents expired so we are seeing a lot of new programs featuring clear aligners. One of the more highly marketed one claims that you can take the impressions in your own home, submit them to their home office, and then get a set of aligners to start using—all without ever having to visit a dentist or orthodontist. There are several problems with this. One is getting accurate impressions. While we use a 3-D scanner, these programs rely on the patients being able to get accurate impressions of their own mouths, using the same old-fashioned goopy stuff that everyone always hated. I have staff members who have been taking impressions for years, and they still don't get it right all the time. Having an entire treatment plan based on the molds taken by a novice of his or her own mouth sounds like a recipe for disaster—or certainly, a less than optimal outcome.

A couple of the programs are now having their scanning centers in and around larger cities. So, they'll have a storefront where you can go in and get a 3-D scan, like we do in our office. Once you have the scan, it's submitted to a reviewer, who decides if you're a candidate or not for the do-it-at-home program. So, they never examine you. They never assess the health of your gums. They never assess the health of your jaw. They just look to see if you have crooked teeth. If you're a candidate, they ship the aligners out to you, without any supervision.

As I said before, it's very easy to straighten teeth. Anyone can do it, with a little bit of training. But when you straighten the teeth, it can dramatically affect your bite. For example, as you age, the most common place to get crowding is in your lower front teeth. Normally, when there's crowding in your lower front teeth, the top front teeth come right down on top of them. So, if you straighten the lower front teeth, if you push them out, then it pushes against the top teeth, and you've completely changed your bite.

It's also a myth that these programs are always cheaper than going to an experienced, hands-on orthodontist. They charge around $2,000. An orthodontist treating the same minor problem will charge about the same. In fact, this brings us to our next myth.

MYTH: **Orthodontics is always expensive, costing at least $5,000 to $6,000 every time.**

REALITY: **The cost of braces depends on the difficulty of the case, and many cases aren't that difficult.**

The cost of treatment for minor cases can be as low as $2,000. More difficult cases will cost more. So, if there is a minor crowding problem that is only going to take four or five months to correct, it's not going to cost $5,000 or $6,500; it's going to be closer to $2,000, or $2,500, which is about the fee that you'd pay for those at-home programs.

So, would you rather pay $2,000 for Smile Direct Club—where you have no supervision and you do it all yourself and you never see an orthodontist—or pay about the same amount of money and get professional supervision? In addition, patients should look at orthodontics as an investment. If you have a more involved case, plan on the orthodontic fee being between $5,000 or $6,500. But again, you are investing in a smile you will have for decades. How much did you pay for your car, and how long did that last?

MYTH: **If I go to an orthodontist as an adult, I need to be prepared for a full set of braces, no matter how minor my problem.**

REALITY: **As an adult, you are in control. If you just want to do partial treatment to make your smile look good, you can.**

When we deal with children, we aim to correct everything—teeth, bite and anything else affecting the teeth—because we are setting them up to have great teeth for a lifetime. But adults often don't want or need the Cadillac of treatment. They just want their smile to look better. They don't care if their back teeth are a bit crooked, or if their bite isn't perfect. They have lived with it for years. If that's all they want, we can oblige. In cases like that, we might use just partial braces on top and be done in a few months. As an informed adult, you have a greater say in your treatment plan.

MYTH: **If I had braces as a child, I'll never need them again.**

REALITY: **Teeth tend to shift as we age, so many adults are going back to clear aligners or braces to have minor crowding adjusted.**

Whether you'll need (or want) additional treatment as an adult is partly dependent on how well you've taken care of your teeth since you had braces. If you've continued to wear your retainer over the years, the likelihood of shifting is reduced. But frankly, it's only been in the past few years that orthodontists pushed the idea that retainers should be worn for a lifetime. Back in the day, orthodontists recommended that they be worn just for a couple of years. If the patient lost the retainer (a really common occurrence), it wasn't replaced. Now, we always recommend long-term retainer wear. So, if you continue to wear the retainers, the teeth should stay straight. But teeth are no different than any other part of the body; they change with age. If you've ever accidentally bitten your cheek or your finger, you know how much force there is in your bite. Imagine what that force must do to each individual tooth when they are used for hundreds of thousands of bites throughout your lifetime. The changes to your teeth occur over time because of the force they endure. A person's face and jaw can continue to grow well into their twenties and sometimes thirties, and this can cause teeth to shift. Your teeth are really in a dynamic state.

I always tell patients, "You know, when we put your teeth in the final position, it's not like we're putting them in bricks and mortar. They cannot be stiff. They have to move, they have to function, and they have to have a little give so you don't break your teeth. So, there's always that natural give to the teeth, and sometimes that can cause shifting later on."

That means, sometimes you get into your forties or fifties and just need get a little tune-up. Once you begin to see shifting or crowding, it's only going to get worse. It's like an arch in a building; you loosen one brick and the other bricks tend to collapse. Same thing with the mouth. If one tooth begins to move out of place, others follow suit. If you can catch it early, it can save you a lot of money and a lot of time in braces or aligners.

This type of tune-up is perfect for Invisalign or SureSmile

aligners. It's almost like those systems were made just for middle-agers who want their teenage teeth back.

MYTH: **If I have missing teeth or crowns, I can't have orthodontic treatment.**

REALITY: **Yes, you can.**

In fact, I often work closely with family dentists to align the teeth better, so they can replace missing teeth correctly.

MYTH: **I can't get braces if I have gum disease.**

REALITY: **This one is partly true.**

We don't put braces on people with active gum or bone disease, but once it's been taken care of by their dentist or periodontist, we can treat them just like any other case. It's actually pretty common to treat people who have had gum disease, but now have it under control. When patients have gum disease, the bone weakens, and the teeth tend to spread. We can use braces to close the gaps and get their smile back. We don't want to put braces on where there's an active periodontal infection, but once that's been treated, yes, you can certainly have orthodontic treatment to correct your problems.

MYTH: **I should get my wisdom teeth removed to prevent crowding.**

REALITY: **There are many, many studies that show this is a myth, but I still hear it all the time.**

There's no correlation between wisdom teeth and crowding. Now, are there other reasons to have wisdom teeth out? Yes. If they're angled, they can affect the tooth in front of them. They can be cystic or infected. There are many, many reasons to legitimately have wisdom teeth out. But to have wisdom teeth out for the sole purpose of, "Oh, it's going to keep my teeth from crowding later." That's been disproven.

A Great Smile to Last Forever

Don't cry because it's over,
smile because it just happened.
DR. SEUSS

The stories I've shared in this book are just the tip of the iceberg. I've seen thousands of children and adults walk out of my office with huge smiles on their faces. Some came in with just minor problems, others were more difficult. They left happy and confident that they could now face the world with the confidence a great smile brings. Knowing I had something to do with how they feel makes my day every time.

We've all heard that beauty is only skin deep, or you can't judge a book by its cover, but truth is, we make quick judgments based on perceptions all the time. One of the most universal biases is toward pleasant-looking people. Straight, white teeth and a welcoming smile are one of the first things we see when we meet people, and we therefore make an instant judgment based on that smile. If that smile is pleasant, the person is perceived as nice, intelligent—someone I'd like to hang out with. The converse is also true.

The benefits of orthodontic care are not just cosmetic. Straight teeth are easier to clean and better anchored, meaning less gum and bone disease, fewer lost teeth and possibly less heart disease and strokes.

It's now possible for everyone to have straight, healthy teeth, and a beautiful smile. And I do mean everyone. Whether you are in middle school or middle-aged, whether you are just learning to read or just recently retired from a job you held for more than forty years, you are a candidate for braces or clear aligners.

There is no reason not to investigate orthodontic treatment. Advances in technology have made the processes easier and shorter than in the past. Nonvisible options, whether they be clear aligners, lingual braces or ceramic, have made orthodontic treatment more acceptable to more and more people.

With all the insurance, FSA and in-house payment plans, the cost of braces can usually be worked into anyone's budget in combination with our in-house payment plans. For those who truly can't afford braces, I and other orthodontists donate countless hours to pro bono work. This pro bono work is close to my heart, and the ability to use my free time to help others is one of the great advantages of running my own practice. Two services that you can contact and that we work with are Smiles Changes Lives and the American Association of Orthodontist Donated Services. You can look them up on the web.

Finally, myself and my staff have a super rewarding job. We see it every day. How cool is it that we can help you get the smile you've always wanted for yourself or your child?

FAQ About Orthodontics

What is orthodontics?

Orthodontics is a specialized form of dentistry focusing on the diagnosis, prevention, and treatment of dental and facial abnormalities. (See Chapter 1 for additional information.)

What is an orthodontist?

An orthodontist is a dental specialist who has received two to three years of additional training and experience beyond the four years of dental school. Your orthodontist is able to straighten teeth, correct misaligned jaw structure, and improve the appearance of your smile. (See Chapters 1 and 2 for additional information.)

How do I know my orthodontic provider is an orthodontist?

Just ask this simple question: "Are you a board-certified orthodontist who has two to three years of additional orthodontic training beyond dental school?"

What's the best age to visit the orthodontist?

If you want to improve the look and feel of your smile, then any age can be a great age to see the orthodontist. I recommend that children first visit an orthodontist around the age of seven; however, orthodontic treatment is not exclusive to children and teens, with about one in every three orthodontic patients being over the age of twenty-one. Whether you're considering treatment for yourself or for a child, any time is a good time to visit the orthodontist. I've treated patients as young as three and as old as eighty-three. (See Chapter 3 for additional information.)

Can you ever be too old to visit an orthodontist?

No. As long as your teeth, gums and jaw bone are healthy, you are a candidate for orthodontic care. Teeth can be moved at any age. (See Chapter 4 for additional information.)

What are braces?

Standard braces consist of a wire attached to your teeth via small metal brackets on each tooth. The wire exerts pressure that gently moves the teeth into position. Clear aligners, such as Invisalign and SureSmile aligners, use flexible, clear plastic trays that fit completely over the teeth. There are several different types of braces to choose from, including: ceramic braces, lingual braces, and traditional metal braces, as well as systems, such as SureSmile, that accelerate treatment and enhance the precision of braces. (See Chapter 5 for additional information.)

If I get braces, how long do I have to wear them?

The amount of time spent in braces will vary depending on the individual patient, because every smile responds differently to treatment. In my office, the average treatment plan runs about sixteen months. Some minor problems might be in and out of braces in just four or five months, while more complicated cases can take up to two years. (See Chapter 6 for additional information.)

Do braces hurt?

Braces do not often hurt, though you may feel a small amount of soreness for a couple days as your teeth, gums, cheeks, and mouth get used to your new braces. (See Chapters 6 and 7 for additional information.)

How can I take care of my teeth if I'm wearing braces or a retainer?

Brushing is the foundation for all good dental hygiene. If you do nothing else, remember to brush after every meal. In addition, continue to see your dentist at least every six months for professional cleanings. (See Chapter 7 for additional information.)

Do I need to brush my teeth more often if I have braces?

With braces, you should brush your teeth at least three times a day—preferably right after you eat—to keep your teeth, gums, and mouth healthy and plaque free. Brushing regularly will help remove any food that may be caught between the braces. (See Chapter 7 for additional information.)

If I have braces, do I still need dental checkups every six months?

Yes! In fact, it's even more important that patients receiving orthodontic treatment visit their dentist regularly. With braces, food may be caught in places that your toothbrush can't reach. This causes bacteria to build up that can lead to cavities, gingivitis, and gum disease. Your dentist will work closely with your orthodontist to make sure that your teeth stay clean and healthy while wearing braces. (See Chapter 7 for additional information.)

Will my braces interfere with activities like sports, playing an instrument, or singing?

Playing an instrument or a contact sport may require some adjustment when you first get your braces, but wearing braces will not stop you from participating in any of your school activities. If you play a contact sport, it is recommended that you wear a mouth guard to protect your braces or appliance. (See Chapter 7 for additional information.)

How do I schedule my first appointment?

Simply call our practice—(815) 436-2959! Our front desk staff will be happy to help schedule your next appointment at your convenience. If you are a new patient or have been referred to our practice, please let us know and we will provide you with all of the information you need. You can visit our website to get more information— https://www.stevemortho.com.